MULTIPLE SCLEROSIS

Multiple Sclerosis

*A Positive Approach
to Living with MS*

CHRIS McLAUGHLIN

Editorial Consultant:
Dr Alexander Burnfield

BLOOMSBURY

First published 1997
Bloomsbury Publishing Plc, 38 Soho Square, London W1V 5DF
Copyright © 1997 Chris McLaughlin
The moral right of the author has been asserted
A copy of the CIP entry for this book is available from the British Library

ISBN 0 7475 2820 9

10 9 8 7 6 5 4 3 2 1

Jacket design by AB3
Typeset by Hewer Text Composition Services, Edinburgh
Printed in Great Britain by Cox & Wyman Ltd, Reading

ACKNOWLEDGEMENTS

First I must warmly thank all the people with MS who gave me so many valuable insights into their lives and especially Helena Jeffs who introduced me to many of them. Isabelle Rickard of Bloomsbury Publishing first suggested that I might take the project on and gave me her time and support well beyond the call of duty. Thanks are also due to Ruth Carlyle and her colleagues at the MS Society for their endless patience in providing information and answering my questions. I received a great deal of useful material from many other organizations and much help from their staff which I greatly appreciated. I would particularly like to thank Christine Jones of the MS (Research) Charitable Trust who also volunteered to read the manuscript and gave me valuable advice.

Many other people, including doctors and other health professionals, were generous with their time and expertise and I am grateful to every one of them.

CONTENTS

FOREWORD

'In an attempt to reduce the chaos which enters their lives with MS, many people try to find patterns or explanations for what is happening to them.'

This book sets out to help with finding patterns and explaining the unpredictable and often capricious effects of MS for people who are affected by it – not only the person diagnosed with the disease, but the people closest to them. Put a dozen people with MS in a room together, and you could easily assume that you were looking at a dozen different diseases. *Multiple Sclerosis* illustrates this through the voices of a group of people who recount their experience of different ways of learning to live with MS, with the conviction that comes only from a personal encounter. For so long, the medical assumption about MS has been that nothing could be done about it, but this group of witnesses shows that much can be done about it, both with and without medical help. Personal motivation and good information, support from friends, family or professionals, all make it possible to strike a truce with MS at worst, and even to surmount it at best.

Chris McLaughlin has written a genuinely comprehensive book about living with MS, which is up to date at the time of going to print. It is an encouraging sign of how rapidly things are changing that many of the advances and ideas she sees on the horizon are likely to be fact or history by the time the book reaches the shops. The new drugs, the alternative therapies, the personal discoveries, are discussed without prejudice or dogma. By definition, people with MS are adults and this book treats them as such, offering information and summarizing the evidence for readers to weigh and then reach their own conclusions. In the absence of clear explanations from scientists or of treatment from doctors, self-management has been the route that many people with MS have taken. This is a travel guide to MS that points out the small things as well as the most prominent, signposts other information sources, and invites travellers to choose for themselves what they will visit and where they will stay.

Like a travel guide, this is not a book that must be read from cover to cover immediately, packed though it is with information and ideas. There is much to be said about MS that is true at any one time for only a proportion of people; for many there is little point in contemplating what may not affect them until and unless they need to do so. But as symptoms come and go, this is a book to be brought out again for a direct and truthful account of different aspects of MS. The distinctive feature of the condition is its unpredictability, which often makes planning difficult, sometimes impossible. *Multiple Sclerosis* is a companion that will help to place the new and unexpected, and to make sense of the changing landscape as the individual journey with MS unfolds.

Peter Cardy
Chief Executive, Multiple Sclerosis Society of Great Britain and Northern Ireland

INTRODUCTION

This book was originally to have been written by my friend and colleague Jenny Glew. She found out that she had MS in 1991, a few months after a mastectomy operation following the return of breast cancer. As a health and consumer journalist, Jenny set herself to find out as much as she could about MS, just as she had done with the breast cancer which first struck in 1988. With the benefit of hindsight and her newly acquired knowledge, she realized that she had probably had the first symptoms of MS at the age of nineteen. Whether any of her doctors had ever suspected the real reason for her intermittent symptoms was to remain a mystery as her medical notes had disappeared.

Jenny was determined that MS should interfere as little as possible with her busy family, social and working life and she continued to pack in enough activity to exhaust a healthy person. Her mobility was becoming seriously limited, but she still made it up the two flights of stairs to the office we had shared for many years, using the pauses to catch up on gossip with everyone else in the building. She explored every available treatment option and, as well as taking orthodox drugs, she tried a range of complementary therapies. By now her MS was progressive, but she felt that she gained a lot from the therapists who treated her, especially her reflexologist. She also enjoyed her regular sessions of hyperbaric oxygen at her local MS therapy centre where, typically, she made a host of new friends. Like everyone, Jenny had her black moments, but she never lost her natural talent for seeing the funny side of life.

She was keen to share what she had learned about MS with others, and wrote articles about it just as she'd always written from her own experience on everything from motherhood to breast cancer. She had planned to start writing this book in the summer of 1995, but in May she was admitted to hospital for tests to try and identify the source of a new symptom – severe back pain.

Well-informed as she was, Jenny was less shocked than the rest of us to learn that it was caused not by MS but by the return of cancer, this time in her spine. During her two months as an inpatient in various hospitals, Jenny's bed was constantly surrounded by family, friends and colleagues talking, sharing her chocolates and laughing. When I visited her for the last time at the Margaret Centre at Whipps Cross Hospital in Essex, we took her laptop computer to a vacant office she persuaded staff to lend us and worked on an article. She was planning to go home soon and start this book. Two days later, she had slipped into sudden and unexpected unconsciousness from which she never emerged.

While the fact that her illness was incurable was no secret, her sudden death hit everyone who knew her very hard. She was one of those exceptional individuals everyone warmed to instantly. Somehow she made people feel better for just being with her or even talking to her on the phone and her death left a gap in the lives of us all. This is not the book Jenny would have written but it does reflect a lot of what I learned from knowing her. She was a very special person.

MS and You

In an ideal world, everyone with MS should have their own personalized version of this book, tailored to their individual needs and their MS. No two people are ever affected in exactly the same way, and every individual's reaction will be different. Every aspect of your life will be relevant to how you deal with MS – whether it's your personality, the course your condition takes, your support network, financial and work situations, family commitments and so on.

I hope you will pick and choose amongst all the information offered here to find the parts that are of use to you personally.

In many of the chapters, you will find liberally scattered quotes outlining the experiences of people who have MS. In sharing their stories and talking to many of them, I was constantly reminded of the need to avoid generalizations about the reality of MS. There is, of course, no single answer to the problems which may be raised when you are having to live with it. For some people, even the possibility of a cure for the condition did not feature on their list of real concerns. For others, it was the only thing which they could see making their lives better. In between are a wide range of opinions and experiences which may or may not strike a chord with individual readers.

Rather than write a mini-biography every time I included a quote from one of these people, I have just used their names in the text. For those of you who would like to know a little more about them, here is a brief introduction, in no particular order.

WHO'S WHO

William Aged twenty-nine, his MS was diagnosed in 1994. He is still able to work and, following a successfully treated bout of depression after his first attack, is now reasonably well. He feels that MS has not affected his relationship with his partner at all.

Frances Aged forty-two, her MS was diagnosed in 1988. She has had to give up working as a hospital nurse and suffers from fatigue and has other symptoms. She has married since learning of her diagnosis but has no children.

Graeme Aged thirty-two, his MS was diagnosed in 1991. He experiences frequent relapses and exacerbations which led him to give up his job as a social worker. Having had a rest, he would now like to work again, but feels prospective employers are wary of him. He and his partner have a two-year-old son.

Chloe Aged twenty-eight, her MS was diagnosed in 1994. At the moment, many of her symptoms are 'invisible', and this makes her job in the media even more stressful. Fatigue and sometimes problems with speech and mental acuity are especially difficult. She has recently separated from her partner, but doubts that her MS was a factor in the break-up.

Janet Aged forty-one, her MS was diagnosed in 1988. Although she had experienced symptoms for several years, she was 'stunned' by the diagnosis. She is unable to work and getting out is difficult. She says she has a marvellous relationship with her partner who knew all about her MS when they met five years ago.

Hazel Aged sixty-one, her MS was diagnosed in 1952. Since then, she has led a very full life with the support of her husband and family. At one time, she was treated (unsuccessfully) with various poisons, including arsenic, belladonna and snake venom! She has had attacks and remissions over the years and her mobility is now limited. She has three grown-up children who were all academically very successful.

Valerie Aged forty-seven, her MS was diagnosed in 1986. She now suffers from muscle pain and seizures and fatigue and had to give up her job in a teaching hospital eight years ago. Her partner, who is a doctor, could not cope with her condition and they parted. She considers herself to be 'philosophical but not accepting' about her MS.

Martin Aged thirty-eight, his MS was diagnosed in 1989. He has experienced symptoms for seventeen years but was only told the truth after persistently pressing for it. His symptoms have got progressively but slowly worse, although he is still able to work as a police officer. He is recently divorced and has two young sons.

Helena Aged thirty-four, her MS was diagnosed in 1994. She had had symptoms since the age of fourteen and suspected MS but was wrongly diagnosed on several occasions. She still works four days a week as a researcher, but finds fatigue a problem and her limited mobility prevents her from going to the canteen with colleagues! Her original partner left 'in horror', but she now has a new and happy relationship.

Ann Aged thirty-five, her MS was diagnosed in 1994. Her main symptoms – numbness in the hands and tingling in the hands and feet – are constant, and she experiences a lot of fatigue, especially in hot weather. She is learning to 'pace herself' and to work out her priorities instead of saying yes to everyone and everything.

Sarah Aged thirty, her MS was diagnosed in 1994. Her main symptom now is numbness, although she has had several attacks since 1978 when she was twelve years old. She was distraught at the diagnosis initially, but now feels that she has been lucky as her symptoms are relatively mild. She says her husband is 'comfortable' with her MS, and as they have two small boys, she is determined to stay strong.

Sue Aged forty-seven, her MS was diagnosed in 1989. Her first attack was five years earlier, and she strongly suspected what was wrong as her father and one of his sisters had MS. She now has a slow progression of her symptoms with the occasional relapse, which always occurs in the first quarter of the year. After initially cutting her hours, she left her job but is involved in voluntary work.

Lizzy Aged forty-four, her MS was diagnosed in 1992. She first had symptoms in 1987, and asked her doctor in 1989 whether it was MS. Her MS is progressive 'just like being on a slide' and she does not have relapses as such. She has a good relationship with her boyfriend, whom she met after being diagnosed. Physiotherapy and a range of complementary therapies have been more help than orthodox medicine.

Paul Aged forty-three, his MS was diagnosed in 1994. His symptoms have got slightly worse since then but he is still able to commute to work. Although relatively unaffected physically, he is concerned that his fear that 'time may be running out' may be affecting his attitude to life in general and his marriage in particular. He and his wife have one teenage son.

Robin Aged thirty-seven, his MS was diagnosed in 1985. Intention tremor and fatigue have forced him to give up climbing and curtail other sporting activities and he retired from his job in engineering four years ago. He believes that attitude is all-important: 'A combination of my strong Christian faith and sheer bloody mindedness gets me through most situations.'

You will also see quite a lot of comments from Jenny who was to have been the author of this book (see page 1). The quotations are mostly taken from Jenny's own writing about her MS which she did both for publication and for herself. A few also come from conversations we had over the years or from experiences which we shared.

chapter one

WHAT IS MS?

For anyone who has multiple sclerosis, the major concern is what impact MS will have on you personally, on your well-being and way of life. Much of the rest of this book will be devoted to considering this aspect. First, however, we need to understand the underlying disease process – what is actually happening inside your body to cause this strange pattern of symptoms.

The Disease Process

MS attacks the central nervous system (or CNS) – that is, the brain and spinal cord. The CNS is made up of billions of nerve cells (grey matter) linked together by fibres of varying length which run down from the brain via the spinal cord to connect with other nerves all over the body. This complex network is the medium through which the brain sends messages to and receives messages back from all parts of your body. The way each nerve is constructed is often compared to an electric cable. The inner part (or axon) corresponding to the wire is enclosed in a protective layer of fatty insulation like the plastic coating on a cable. This layer is called the myelin sheath. It is made up of various proteins and fats and is often referred to as 'white matter'.

The nerves comprising this vital 'control centre' are constantly coated in a fluid called cerebro-spinal fluid to enable the CNS to function properly. Additional protection is provided by a membrane known as the blood-brain barrier. Its purpose is to limit access by undesirable substances dissolved in the bloodstream to the CNS itself. In people with MS, this filter mechanism loses some of its effectiveness, so the CNS becomes vulnerable to attack. No one yet understands why this change occurs, but the evidence points to MS being what's called an autoimmune disease. For some reason, elements of the body's immune system go awry and, in effect, start a civil war. Normally, the immune system protects the body against disease by destroying invaders such as bacteria and viruses but in MS, it appears to turn on itself and attack the myelin sheath. The result is that the tissue becomes inflamed and, if the attack continues, a small segment of the sheath is destroyed. In the areas where the sheath has been damaged (known as plaques or lesions), scar tissue (or sclerosis) develops and interferes with the smooth transmission of impulses travelling along the nerve to and from the brain. Since the messages can no longer be transmitted efficiently along this particular pathway, they can't fulfil their task of controlling movement or responding to sensation as well as they should.

This process, known as demyelination, may occur in one or more locations within the CNS. Exactly what symptoms the person gets and how severe they are will depend on which nerves are affected and how badly. Part of the clinical definition of MS is that such attacks not only take place in different parts of the CNS but also at different times. In between, the symptoms may subside or even disappear completely, sometimes for long periods. When another bout of inflammation sets in, the symptoms may be different if a different part of the myelin sheath is targeted. As you are probably already aware, the way MS affects you is unique to you and no other individual will experience it in exactly the same way. One of the hardest things to accept about this condition is that no one can tell what course it will take in the weeks, months or even years after diagnosis. Until we have direct experience of it, either ourselves or from someone close to us, most of us know only the classic image of the person with MS in a wheelchair who has become seriously disabled by the disease, sometimes in a relatively short time. In fact, the minority of people – around 20 per cent – who are this profoundly affected are at one end of a very broad spectrum. At the other are people who have only very mild symptoms or have one attack and then no further symptoms at all. This group is also estimated to make up around 20 per cent of all people with MS. In between these two poles are people who experience a variety of symptoms which may come and go or only worsen very slowly, but who nevertheless manage to get round the difficulties without any dramatic disruption to their lives for many years. In some cases, the pattern eventually changes so that they start to experience increasing disability without periods of noticeable remission.

The range of possible symptoms is wide (as we will see on page 19) and depends on exactly which nerves are affected. They may be located in any part of the CNS and be responsible for transmitting different kinds of messages. The motor nerves specialize in controlling movement of all kinds; the sensory nerves deal with feeling and sensation and the optic nerves form the link between eyes and brain. They all work in conjunction with the complex network of nerves feeding instructions and information from all parts of the body to and from the brain.

The exact points at which scarring occurs seem to be significant. On the one hand, a relatively small number of plaques – on an optic nerve or a particular spot in the brain, for example – can have severe repercussions in terms of disability. On the other hand, extensive scarring of the myelin sheath is sometimes revealed during postmortem examinations of people who had few or no MS symptoms and died of some other illness. Areas of scarring can be seen through a test called Magnetic Resonance Imaging (or MRI) which uses a magnetic field to take detailed pictures of the brain and spinal cord. In some people, the correlation between damage visible from an MRI scan and actual symptoms seems not to be very close. In other words, they do not always have the symptoms which would be expected, or conversely experience problems in areas which the MRI findings would not have predicted.

This is one of the reasons why your experience of MS will differ from everyone else's. In fact it is almost impossible to exaggerate the degree of variability in the way different people experience the condition. This applies not only between one person and another, but also in a single individual over time. However, some of the differences are likely to depend on which form of the condition you have. In broad terms, there are usually said to be two major categories: relapsing-remitting and progressive. In addition, people in the latter group are further sub-divided into those who have primary progressive and secondary progressive MS. However, the distinction is not always clear-cut and is based purely on the pattern of symptoms shown by the individual. There are no tests which can tell you which group you belong to.

In theory, the difference is that people with relapsing-remitting MS will have intervals when their symptoms abate or even disappear, while those in the other group have no such relief. In practice, however, it is not always easy to assign any one person to a specific category, even though the distinction holds true in general. In a minority of people, MS seems to take the progressive form from the outset; this is known as primary progressive MS and is comparatively rare, affecting some 15 per cent of people. Others may have intervals of remission lasting for several years between attacks before their symptoms seem to take a more permanent hold. This group are then said to have developed secondary progressive MS and this applies to about 40 per cent of people with the condition.

While these classifications are undoubtedly meaningful in overall terms, they may not be of much help to the individual person with MS. If you have MS, you will almost certainly have had a range of symptoms which bothered you for some time before the condition was diagnosed. They may have been minor or more serious and been with you for long periods or have eased or even disappeared after a while. It's likely that you – and possibly your doctor too – initially ascribed them to other causes or you may have managed to dismiss them as insignificant and not worth investigating.

In about a fifth of all people with MS, the condition remains relatively benign. While living with MS is never easy, for people who fall into this category it is possible to overcome the problems without the need to make dramatic changes to their former lifestyle. They may have one or two attacks from which they appear to recover completely so that the illness causes no further symptoms.

The biggest group are those who go through phases when the disease is active and they develop new symptoms or experience a recurrence of old ones. These relapses can last anything from minutes to months and occur very close together or after quite long intervals. After the flare-up subsides, the symptoms may disappear, but often they leave the person somewhat more badly affected than they were before.

When the condition takes the progressive form, there are usually few or no periods when the person is symptom-free, although they may remain relatively stable for months or even years. But, as is inevitably the case with MS, there are exceptions even to this rule, and some people do experience remissions from time to time.

Researchers who have studied the course of the disease in thousands of individuals have analysed factors which may be significant in predicting future developments. It has been suggested, for example, that people whose MS begins before the age of forty and whose first symptom is visual disturbance caused by inflammation of the optic nerve are relatively unlikely to become severely disabled. This may also be the case if there is a long period of remission following the first attack. On the other hand, those who are thought to have developed the primary progressive form later in life may have quite serious problems with their bladder and with mobility, but find that their arms and their cognitive abilities remain relatively unaffected. There is also evidence that the degree of disability a person is experiencing five years after the onset of MS may be relevant. The fewer problems present at this stage, the better the outlook. It hardly needs saying, however, that individuals can and do frequently defy these predictions!

This unpredictability is what many people find the hardest thing to bear. We have mostly come to take it for granted that while medical science can't cure all diseases, it can usually give us some idea of what the future holds. Even if the prognosis is bad, at least we can try to come to terms with it and prepare ourselves for what may lie ahead. Sadly, even this Job's comforter is not on offer to people with MS, or not yet anyway. However, this very uncertainty does contain some ray of hope because it means that while no one can say when or if the symptoms will get worse, neither can they say that they won't get better.

In some way that's not yet understood, the central nervous system possesses the ability to heal itself. Damaged nerve fibres can and do regrow and remyelination of scarred parts of the myelin sheath does occur. When and why this recovery takes place is not clear so far, but the fact that it happens at all leaves open the possibility of temporary or even permanent remission.

One thing that is immediately clear from all this is that while everyone with MS shares the same underlying disease process – the malfunction of parts of the central nervous system due to demyelination – they are likely to differ from one another in many important respects. The range of possible symptoms and their severity, duration and persistence are different for everyone. The way you deal with having the illness will also be unique to you and will have a bearing on how you are affected by it.

Many people will say that there are two distinct stages in understanding a diagnosis of MS. Some make a point of learning as much as they can about what exactly goes wrong in their bodies as a result of the disease, while others are content with a less detailed picture. Either way, you are then faced with the prospect of understanding your MS and

13

finding out how you can live with the particular problems it brings for you. And, of course, this process may well have to be gone through more than once. Just when you think you've got it worked out, the disease may suddenly manifest itself in a different way, and you have to go through the whole process of adjustment all over again.

William: *'Before my MS was diagnosed in July 1994, I had severe pain in my face, tinnitus [ringing and other noises in the ears], visual difficulties, pins and needles in my arms and legs and severe lack of coordination in my fingers – so I couldn't use push button phones, for example, and kept dropping cups of coffee and tea. After three to four months, all the symptoms cleared up and I've had no problems since. I'm just hoping that this period of remission will last!'*

Graeme: *'At the time of diagnosis, I had paralysis down the right side of my body. Since then, over the last five years, I've had blurred vision, weakness, tiredness and severe headaches. All these come and go over the year, and can last from a couple of days to a couple of months.'*

Sue: *'I had symptoms from 1984, and my first relapse in 1986 before being diagnosed in 1989. Early on, I had fluctuating symptoms – numbness, cold patches on my skin and a feeling of a stone in my shoe. The first attack brought foot drop, fatigue and an inability to walk more than 200 metres. Then there was complete remission and I was back to playing sports. Thereafter, I had occasional relapses followed by partial remission and gradual lessening of control. I have some incontinence, with bladder urgency and minimal bowel control. Now it seems to be a slow progression with the occasional relapse. My walking is very limited, speech and* *memory are affected and I have constant fatigue. The relapses last around one or two months, then I return to 80 per cent of my previous level.'*

Martin: *'For seventeen years I've had various symptoms: numbness, pins and needles, unsteady balance, occasional slurred speech, heavy legs, occasional sexual impotence, clumsiness, weakness in various muscles and more. In 1981, I became almost blind in my left eye overnight. My sight returned over several weeks, though the damage was never fully repaired. Now it is much improved, though for a long time it felt as though I were looking through mosquito netting. I have become gradually worse – weaker and my walking is less efficient – but the progression seems very slow.'*

Who gets MS?

There are approximately 85,000 people in the UK who have been diagnosed as having MS and they are more likely to be women than men in a proportion of three to two. Although you can experience the first symptoms at almost any age, the most common time for the condition to be diagnosed is in the late twenties or early thirties. It used to be said that MS never struck before the age of fifteen or so, but it is now known that children can be affected too, although this is relatively unusual. At the other end of the spectrum, some people only discover they have MS in their late fifties.

The picture of who gets MS and when is being redrawn

largely in response to improved techniques of diagnosis which mean that it can now be identified in many people who previously would not have known what was causing their symptoms. For example, it was once thought that people born and brought up in China or Japan rarely or never developed the condition, but cases are increasingly being discovered in these and other areas where it was previously unrecognized.

Nevertheless, geography still seems to play some part in determining who gets MS. It is much more common in people who live in countries with a temperate climate. In other words, the further away from the Equator you live, the higher your risk of developing MS. Countries lying between 40 and 60 degrees of latitude are those with the highest risk. In addition, some regions seem to have a particularly high incidence of the disease. The numbers of people affected are relatively larger in northern Europe, especially Scotland and Scandinavia. And it's apparently not just a question of where you live now, but rather where you were born and brought up. If you move from a country with a tropical climate to one with a temperate climate (or vice versa) before you reach puberty, you acquire the same risk of developing MS as people who've always lived in your new country. Making the same move later (in your mid-teens onwards) will mean your risk remains the same as that faced by people in the country you left. So, for example, a two-year-old whose family moved from Mombasa to London or from Sri Lanka to Auckland would face an increased risk of developing MS while his sixteen-year-old sister would not. This obviously implies that something in the environment is affecting the level of risk, although, equally obviously, it isn't the whole story. It's thought that the higher incidence of MS in countries such as Scotland and Scandinavia is probably due to some inherent vulnerability shared by many of the inhabitants in those areas.

All these variations are not surprising, bearing in mind what is known about the causes of MS. It seems that several factors may have to be combined in any one individual in order for them to develop the disease. The first is some sort of genetic susceptibility. Although it is not a directly inherited condition passed on in the genes like cystic fibrosis or Duchenne muscular dystrophy, there does seem to be some slight family link as there is with diseases such as heart disease, diabetes, osteoporosis and some forms of cancer, for example. In other words, someone who has a parent, brother or sister with the condition has a slightly increased risk of developing it themselves. As we've seen, MS has the characteristics of an autoimmune disease, and this implies that there may be some abnormality in a person's immune system which causes it to target the myelin sheath. It has been shown that certain tissue types are more likely to be found in people who have MS, which may be part of the explanation for their susceptibility to the disease. Researchers have very recently identified a gene which appears to be connected with a predisposition to develop MS, although it is certainly not a gene 'for MS'. Nevertheless, this break-through will open new avenues of research and should contribute greatly to our understanding of MS in due course.

Even in those individuals who are potentially vulnerable to developing MS, however, it appears that something else has to happen to set the process off. The most likely trigger is a virus of some kind. Various possible candidates have been studied, but as yet none has been shown to be involved. It may be that any one of a number of possible viruses could act as a trigger, including common ones such as measles and herpes, which can remain dormant in the body for some years after the initial infection. The possible role of viral infection in MS is the subject of a lot of current research. The problem is to discover whether a virus can somehow disrupt the immune system and initiate the attack on myelin and, if so, why the virus itself is not sought out and destroyed by the body's defence mechanisms.

These and many other gaps in our knowledge about the causes of MS still need to be filled, but in the meantime, we can say something about what doesn't cause it:

- **It's not contagious**. The fact that one or more viruses may be involved does not mean that you can catch MS from someone else. It is not a viral infection like the common cold, for example.
- **It's not a form of mental illness**. Although some people may develop what are called cognitive symptoms (impaired memory or concentration and personality changes, for example), these are caused by physical changes in the way nerve cells function – the same process which causes the other symptoms of MS.
- **It is not a form of brain damage**. At one time, some doctors believed that injury, in particular a blow to the head, could cause the formation of plaques in the brain and thus might be responsible for MS. In fact, studies have now shown that this is not the case and injuries of any kind do not seem to be implicated in causing MS.
- **It is not an inherited condition**. However, as we've seen, there seems to be some genetic component, and the chances of a close relative of someone with MS developing the disease are higher (1–3 in every 100) than those of the rest of the population (1 in 1,000).

  Nevertheless, many other factors play a part, and most people with the condition will have no similarly affected family members.

The symptoms

One of the problems with MS is that it can seem as if every individual who has it has actually got a different disease judging purely on the basis of the symptoms they experience. A further difficulty when it comes to diagnosis is that in the early stages, many of these symptoms are rather ill-defined and don't all occur at the same time. A numb sensation in your feet, tingling in one or more limbs or not being able to see clearly for a short time, for example, can all be dismissed as an inexplicable oddity or put down to some cause which is in reality unrelated. If your doctor is sufficiently alert he or she may suspect MS when you come to the surgery for the second or third time with some minor complaint of this kind. On the other hand, if you or your GP are new to the practice or your notes have disappeared, it may take some time before the connection is made or even suspected. Even when someone does show symptoms that could indicate MS, there are likely to be many other possible explanations which need to be considered first. Many doctors in any case feel a natural reluctance to suggest the possibility of MS to any patient without very good reason, especially while there is no cure or even effective palliative treatment they can offer. For all these reasons, many people have to wait a long time before they are offered tests to investigate whether they may have MS.

Whether you have already been diagnosed or just suspect that you may have MS, it is important to remember that what follows is a list of *possible* symptoms. No one will have all of them, some may only have one or two and all can come and go, maybe to return later, maybe not.

VISUAL PROBLEMS

For many people, some kind of eye symptom is the first indication that something is wrong. Others may experience visual disturbances later on, perhaps during a relapse, and they can be relatively brief or last for many months. They can sometimes affect just one eye or both, take various forms and be severe or almost unnoticeable. They include:

- Blurred vision
- Double vision
- Blind spots (scotomata)
- Pain and discomfort in the eye
- Nystagmus – flickering eyeballs
- Squint

LOSS OF COORDINATION

This can make it very difficult to do all kinds of things – from walking to making a cup of tea. Instead of being smooth and controlled, your movements become erratic and jerky and you become clumsy and more accident-prone. Shaking hand movements can make life particularly difficult and everyday activities like using a knife and fork turn into a major challenge.

POOR BALANCE

Loss of myelin in a certain area of the brain can cause attacks of giddiness or vertigo or make it impossible for you to stand upright when your eyes are shut. Even with them open, you may feel wobbly when you try to stand still. Some people only get dizzy now and again, but for others it is a more long-term problem.

LOSS OF STRENGTH

You may experience localized weakness which makes it difficult to open screw-top bottles for example, or to run or walk upstairs. Some people also have what feels like a more generalized loss of strength so that it's a real effort to drag yourself around or do jobs like mowing the lawn or bed-making.

SENSORY PROBLEMS

Some people say that these are some of the most difficult symptoms to live with because they can be very peculiar and almost impossible to explain to other people. Sometimes it's even hard to believe that they really are symptoms of MS and not all in your mind!

- **Pins and needles**. This is one of the commonest early symptoms and can last for days at a time or even longer.
- **Tingling**. For some people this is an uncomfortable nuisance, but for others the sensation verges on the painful.
- **Numbness**. This is another common early symptom and causes all kinds of difficulties. When your feet are numb it's impossible to walk properly. People often say it feels like they're treading on thick layers of cotton wool or snow or even as though they're floating above the ground. When other parts of your body are affected, you lose your sense of touch and it's difficult to do quite simple tasks using your hands when you have little or no sensation in your fingers.
- **Clamminess**. Hands and feet may feel clammy and some people find their legs are often cold even in warm rooms or weather. The opposite can happen too – sudden sensations of heat and sweatiness which have nothing to do with the external temperature. This may be due to

21

circulation problems, but it can also happen because plaques are interfering with normal transmission of sensory impulses.

- **Heavy limbs**. This is another of those peculiar symptoms which is particularly distressing because it is so ill defined. Other people often find it hard to understand, but it is very real and makes getting around hard work.

FATIGUE

Almost everyone with MS suffers from this at some time and it is enormously frustrating and hard to live with. Anyone who hasn't experienced it may simply think you're feeling tired or, worse still, swinging the lead, but it can knock you flat within minutes and there's no way to resist it. Although it is in part the result of demyelination and directly attributable to MS, the precise reason why it occurs is not well understood. It may be that you are experiencing the effects of what's sometimes called 'silent damage' to the CNS. In other words, where the myelin sheath has become scarred, message transmission is impaired but you only become aware of the consequences of this damage at certain times, say after exertion or when you are fatigued for some other reason. It is thought that MS may have other effects on the brain which contribute towards inducing fatigue and exacerbate the effects of damage to the myelin sheath itself.

Many people find fatigue strikes suddenly without warning when they're in the middle of some ordinary task, but sometimes it can creep up on you slowly. As anyone who's experienced it knows, it is quite unlike normal tiredness and a good night's sleep is usually not sufficient to cure it. It often goes along with a worsening of other symptoms such as weakness and an inability to think or speak clearly and all your senses may seem dulled. Sometimes you may have symptoms which are new to you, which is frightening because it suggests that the MS is getting worse. In fact there is no evidence that this is so and the symptoms should subside as you recover from the bout of fatigue. Some situations seem prone to set off bouts of fatigue for many people, and we will be looking at that aspect in detail in chapter 7.

SPEECH PROBLEMS

When demyelination affects the nerves controlling the muscles used in speaking, the person may have difficulty in communicating clearly. The most common problem, known medically as dysarthria, can make your voice sound weak or inexpressive and some people can't pronounce words as clearly as they once did. A few people with MS develop problems which affect their brain's ability to process language and thus their ability to understand other people and communicate with them, while others know what they want to say but the message can't get through properly to the muscles controlling speech itself.

SWALLOWING DIFFICULTIES

When muscles in your jaw and throat are not working properly, you may have difficulty swallowing food and especially liquids. Sometimes you can feel as if you may choke, which is unpleasant and frightening. Very hot or cold food or drink can exacerbate the problem and so can any tension or trying to rush a meal. Taking your time may make things easier, and it is sometimes helpful to get advice from a dietician about the right kind of diet.

BLADDER AND BOWEL PROBLEMS

Having to empty your bladder frequently and/or without delay is a vexation familiar to a great many people with MS. For some, it's made even worse because mobility problems limit their ability to get to the loo speedily enough when the need arises. Sometimes, despite all the time spent emptying the bladder, it still retains some urine, which as well as making you uncomfortable can encourage infections such as cystitis. Normally, cystitis is more common in women, but both men and women are likely to be affected when they have MS. The prostate gland can act as a reservoir for infection in men and they may need longer courses of treatment to eradicate the bacteria responsible. In fact, bladder problems can be an early symptom of MS which are not recognised as such and put down to infection or some other cause instead.

Incontinence is one of the more distressing symptoms of MS and it's easy to opt out of social activities rather than risk public embarrassment. Occasionally, bowel incontinence may also develop, but this is less common than constipation. There are various drugs which can help with bladder problems as well as various aids to deal with the problem which we will look at in chapter 2. Meanwhile, it may help to know that this kind of symptom often comes and goes and may disappear as suddenly as it began.

MUSCLE STIFFNESS

Changes in your muscle tone can cause your muscles to contract when you don't intend them to, and obviously when your legs are affected walking can be very difficult. Some people find stiffness is the main problem, while for others it's spasms, which can sometimes be painful.

24

PAIN

At one time it was generally thought that pain was not caused by the MS itself, but was either unrelated or due to problems like poor posture or sitting for too long. Now, however, doctors and other health professionals know that people with MS can also experience many different kinds of pain which are directly attributable to CNS damage. These may range from dull aches, burning sensations and sharp pain associated with muscle spasms to pain in the eyes and the acute facial pain caused by trigeminal neuralgia.

SEXUAL DIFFICULTIES

It's hardly surprising that sexual difficulties are not unusual among couples where one of the partners has MS. Apart from the strains imposed on relationships by the illness itself, symptoms such as lack of mobility and fatigue can interfere with a happy sex life. These aspects apart, it's also the case that some individuals may also have symptoms resulting from demyelination which have a direct effect on their sexual response.

- **Men**. It may be difficult or sometimes impossible to get an erection or to stay hard long enough to have sexual intercourse. Some men also notice that the timing and sensation of ejaculation change and occasionally it may bring pain rather than pleasure.
- **Women**. Generally, women need more time to become fully aroused than men, but neurological changes can sometimes make it almost impossible. Some women find loss of sensation a problem, while lack of vaginal lubrication or clitoral engorgement can make sex disappointing or even painful.

Apart from the physical factors which can get in the way of a good sex life, for some couples the situation may be complicated still further by psychological difficulties. When you are struggling to cope with normal life in the face of the problems posed by MS, sex may slip down your list of priorities. You may find it hard to go on seeing yourself as a sexual being or doubt that anyone could still find you attractive. It often takes time for couples to adjust to the changes in their relationship which have been brought about by one partner's illness and this too can have a negative effect on their physical relationship.

PSYCHOLOGICAL CHANGES

You would be a very unusual person indeed if the reality of living with a condition like MS had no effect on you emotionally or psychologically. Depression and mood swings are a common and unsurprising reaction, but it's also possible for psychological symptoms to arise directly from neurological damage. Such cognitive changes are real symptoms of MS just as much as a dragging leg or blurred vision. By no means everyone gets such symptoms, and like the purely physical manifestations, they can come and go at different times.

Research has shown that a person with MS who has most of the CNS lesions in their brain is likely to show greater emotional distress than someone who has most of the lesions in the spinal cord. Depending on the precise area of the brain in which the damage is located, the psychological symptoms may be more dramatic and noticeable.

At one time, little was said publicly about such changes, which tended to be ignored or swept under the carpet. Increasingly, however, there is more openness about what is a particularly distressing aspect of MS for those affected and for their families. It is often hard to recognize what is really happening. For example, if a mother with MS has brain lesions which tend to make her more irritable, she'll be prone to shout at the family more than she used to. However, if her short-term memory is also affected, she may not be aware of how often she is doing it. Even if she is, if her powers of abstract reasoning are not what they were, she may not be able to work out other ways of dealing with the situation. It's easy to see how such a pattern of changes could affect the way a person functions socially, or at work, for example.

Sometimes, neurological changes in the brain can cause behaviour which is very hurtful to other people, even though it is unintentional. The person with MS may lose the ability to understand what effect they are having on those close to them – as if they can no longer empathize with other people's feelings or understand their emotional reactions. For instance, they may decide that it is in their family's best interests to have nothing more to do with them so they can get on with their lives unencumbered. They fail to understand why the family find this attitude hurtful and very upsetting.

- **Memory loss**. Malfunction of short-term memory is quite common and is often a problem in the early stages. You may forget why you've opened the fridge door or find your mind a blank when you try to think of a familiar person's name. Worrying and annoying though this is, it doesn't mean your memory is going entirely or that it is the start of dementia.
- **Loss of concentration**. Some people find they can't keep their mind focused on anything for very long or that their ability to formulate clear plans or think logically seems lower than before. Fatigue can make it impossible to think straight at all for a while, but the feeling often passes as you recover your energy.

- **Personality changes**. Again, these are often more obvious to others than to the person concerned. It can seem as if an individual no longer has any concern or consideration for anyone but themselves, and is constantly irritable or prone to lash out at the slightest (or no) provocation.
- **Depression**. Sometimes this can progress beyond being an emotional reaction to your situation and be the result of plaque formation in a crucial part of your brain responsible for emotional responses.
- **Mood swings**. These are often commented on by the partners of people with MS or those close to them because they can be difficult to live with. The change from calmness to anger, for example, or from being reasonably cheerful to depression can sometimes be dramatic and appear to arise completely out of the blue. It can be especially upsetting when the person with MS seems prone to laugh at inappropriate moments, and this causes distress for those close to them who don't understand why it happens, and for the person him- or herself when they realize it's happening.
- **Euphoria**. The opposite to depression, this was once thought to be quite common among people with MS. Now, however, it is more likely to be seen as one aspect of the loss of control of emotions which can result from neurological damage, and may even mask quite serious underlying depression.

This list is enough to frighten anyone to death, and it is worth stressing again that no one individual will have all of these symptoms, either together or separately. Those which you do have can vary in severity and in duration. Some you may have to find a way of living with, while others disappear of their own accord. Sometimes a symptom may be eased with treatment – medicine, physiotherapy or, very occasionally, surgery – so it is always worth considering this option and discussing it with your doctor.

Many people say it helps to know that some of the more bizarre experiences – such as odd sensory sensations or their memory playing tricks – are recognized as true symptoms of MS and not just the product of their fevered imagination. The so-called 'invisible' systems which, unlike a limp for example, are not immediately obvious to other people are nevertheless still the result of damage to the myelin sheath and subject to the same maddening unpredictability.

We have concentrated here on describing as many of the symptoms as possible, and this obviously conjures up a terrifying prospect. However, while no one can yet offer you treatment which will get rid of them for good, there is a lot that you can do to alleviate their effects and enable you to get on with your life in spite of all that MS may throw at you. We will look at the various options in subsequent chapters.

Getting a diagnosis

As those of you who have already been through it will know, arriving at a diagnosis of MS is usually a slow and somewhat imprecise affair. And occasionally, it can be painfully and unreasonably slow. It's common for people to experience a variety of symptoms for which neither they nor their doctors can find a sensible explanation before the possibility of their being caused by MS is discussed. There are a number of reasons for this delay. When the symptoms are vague and disappear by themselves, they could be unrelated or be caused by a condition other than MS. Some people who've had or still have some of the more classic symptoms, such as visual disturbance, are more likely to be sent for tests quite quickly, but others may have to wait months or even years before reaching this stage.

Even when MS is recognized as a possible diagnosis, it may not be mentioned until or unless you come back with one or more fresh symptoms suggestive of MS. Your doctor will want to wait after the first consultation to see whether you develop any other problem which could indicate that there is damage to a different part of the CNS. A person is not usually said to be suffering from MS unless they have symptoms which indicate damage to at least two different areas of the myelin sheath on at least two separate occasions.

Apart from these clear-cut clinical reasons, many doctors feel there is no point in raising what they see as the spectre of MS before it is absolutely necessary. The justification for this is the desire to protect their patient from having to face the trauma of being told they have MS, especially in view of the fact that the doctor can offer little or nothing by way of treatment. As no one can say how badly any individual may be affected nor even whether they will have further attacks, the theory is that they are best left in blissful ignorance for as long as possible.

The trouble with this well-intentioned approach is that it takes no account of what the individual concerned would prefer. There are undoubtedly some people who are grateful that their doctors kept the suspected diagnosis from them, but there are many others who want to know as much as possible as soon as possible.

However unwelcome the revelation that you may have MS, at least you have some idea of what you're dealing with. Until the possibility is raised for the first time, many people feel that their symptoms have not been taken seriously or accepted as real by other people. The implication is that they were simply suffering from hypochondria or perhaps from some form of mental illness. A woman who was treated for depression for a year, despite complaining of visual disturbances and numbness in her hands and feet, is a fairly typical example of what can happen. Others may have wondered whether their symptoms were caused by some potentially fatal illness such as cancer or a brain tumour. There are too many stories of people with MS who say they had to endure months or years of anxiety or inappropriate treatment before MS was finally diagnosed. An honest and open discussion with your doctor should be the first step towards an understanding of MS and what it will mean for you if the diagnosis is confirmed.

Although what you have told him or her about your past and present symptoms may suggest the possibility of MS to your GP, you will need to be referred to a neurologist for further tests before the diagnosis can be confirmed or otherwise. While there is no one specific test that can give a definitive answer, there are a few which, taken together with your history, can indicate that you do in fact have MS.

- **Medical history**. You'll be asked again to give as many details as you can about your symptoms – when they occurred, how long they lasted and so on plus background information on your general health.
- **Neurological examination**. This is designed to assess whether there are any abnormalities in the way signals are transmitted along your nerve pathways. As well as looking for changes in eye movements, limb co-ordination, weakness, balance and so on, the neurologist will use a hammer to test reflexes or a pinprick test to check sensation. This examination will reveal whether you have any neurological abnormality, but won't shed any light on the probable cause.

31

- **Visual/auditory evoked potentials test**. This is another test to find out whether messages are being passed normally along the nerve pathways, and it can be done in an out-patient clinic. It measures the time taken for the brain to receive a message transmitted in response to a visual or auditory (heard) stimulus by means of small electrodes attached to your head. Normally, the reaction is virtually instantaneous, but when demyelination has occurred there may be a delay because the relevant message is being conducted more slowly. Using this method, the doctor may be able to identify specific areas of scarring, but again, not why they have occurred.

- **Lumbar puncture**. You are given a local anaesthetic to numb your skin, and a small amount of cerebro-spinal fluid (CSF) is drawn out through a needle inserted into your back. This fluid, which surrounds the brain and spinal cord, is then analysed for the presence of antibodies which can occur with MS as well as with other neurological conditions. The test is uncomfortable but not painful. You may have to lie flat for a number of hours afterwards, otherwise you may get a headache. You may also be asked to stay in hospital overnight to give the CSF time to replenish itself.

- **Magnetic resonance imaging (MRI)**. This is the newest of the diagnostic tests and has become more widely available in recent years. It uses a magnetic field to scan the CNS and take detailed pictures of the brain and spinal cord, showing up areas of scarring (sclerosis). While it gives detailed information on the number, size and location of plaques, it may not pick up all of them and can't prove conclusively that MS is the cause of them. However, taken together with a history of your symptoms and the results of other tests, an MRI scan helps to clarify the diagnosis.

Once the information obtained in these various ways has been put together, it should be possible to say whether you do or don't have MS. Normally, the diagnosis will be given to you by a doctor at the hospital, although some people are told by their GPs. How this is done, and what happens next, will depend very much on where you are and who tells you. There are some doctors who appear to believe that once they have given you the news, their job is done. Others will give you the opportunity to discuss the diagnosis and its implications; others feel it is better to do that a little later when you have had time to take the news in properly. Sadly, some doctors seem to have neither natural talent nor adequate training in giving bad news to their patients and come across as cold or uncaring as a result.

Lizzy: *I had been saying there was something seriously wrong with me for three years, with symptoms having started in 1987 and my asking the doctor if I had MS in 1989. My neurologist was on holiday at the time of my tests (in 1992) and I asked the registrar what they were looking for. With a bit of coaxing, she told me it was MS. I was not called to see my neurologist for about two months, which had given me time to investigate the illness a bit. I contacted the MS Society, ARMS and read a couple of books by people who had MS and prepared a double-sided A4 sheet of paper full of questions. The diagnosis itself was a relief – I was not a hypochondriac! The disappointment was in the neurologist's inability to answer my questions which were not taken seriously as some of them were slightly "fringe". He had never heard of anyone with MS being given vitamin B12 injections, which has surprised me even more since then. He did not believe oil of evening primrose did any good but said it would do me no harm. He told me I would be in a wheelchair within five years. When I said I did not have time for that, he said that* *with an attitude like that he would extend it to ten years! The whole time he appeared extremely uncomfortable, which might have been due to the registrar having given me intravenous steroids without his knowledge.'*

Graeme: *'I was given the diagnosis by the consultant neurologist – and I was annoyed, angry, disgusted. It went something like this: "Thanks for letting my students . . . I'm 99.9 per cent sure you have MS . . . We'll start you on steroids . . . and arrange an MRI scan to confirm . . . I've got to run now." He had suggested that I must have suspected that I has MS, but I hadn't a clue. I thought I'd had some sort of stroke. A student nurse brought me some pamphlets and talked with me, but admitted she didn't know anything about MS. However, it was good to talk to her.'*

Should you find yourself in the hands of someone who seems unwilling or unable to give you the information or advice you want, it may be possible to arrange to see another person in the clinic or practice. Alternatively (or additionally), you might like to ring one of the helplines run by organizations like the MS Society or the MS Resource Centre where you can talk over the situation with trained counsellors and find answers to some of your questions.

However, the majority of doctors will be willing to give you time to talk or may be able to put you in touch with other health professionals within the hospital or community.

Paul: *'I have no problems with the way the consultant neurologist broke the news about MS. It was factual and professional. My wife was there, and he showed compassion without emotion. I wasn't given any other specific information, other than about the MS Society. It was left up to me, which is what I prefer.'*

Ann: *'I think the consultant neurologist who gave me the diagnosis did it as well as could reasonably be expected. I was treated as an intelligent, adult person. It is easy to criticize the difficult role of the doctor. I had known rationally that MS was a possibility, but nevertheless the shock of being told was very great.'*

The majority of people with MS are likely to remain in the care of their GP and a neurologist, who will call in other professionals as required. These may well include physiotherapists, urologists (for bladder problems), dieticians and occupational therapists. This can work well, but sometimes it can be a rather hit-and-miss affair.

NEUROREHABILITATION

In some areas, a person with MS may be referred to a consultant in rehabilitation medicine. You may feel this sounds rather unappealing, especially if your MS is not interfering dramatically in your life at present.

Nevertheless, specialists in this field do have something to offer to people with MS. As yet their services are only available in a few centres, but such units are gradually spreading around the country. The specialty is a relatively new one, although rehabilitation centres not specifically devoted to neurological conditions now exist in many hospitals.

Neurorehabilitation concentrates specifically on the needs of people experiencing the consequences of neurological damage. These might include those with spinal and brain injuries and Parkinson's disease as well as people with MS. The idea is to try and minimize each person's symptoms so they they can function as well as possible, given the physical limitations caused by the neurological damage.

At the MS Unit at the Central Middlesex Hospital, the consultant in rehabilitation medicine works with a team including a physiotherapist, a nutritionist, an occupational therapist and a counsellor. Other specialist expertise can be called on if an individual patient needs it. Everyone is offered the opportunity to see each member of the team to discuss and assess their particular problems. Any treatment or other help is tailored to the needs of the individual, with the aim of keeping that person as healthy and independent as possible. One of the big advantages of this kind of approach is that the consultant and his team are able to build up a rounded picture of an individual and their difficulties. They can assess the effectiveness or otherwise of a particular treatment, suggest alternatives and discuss the pros and cons. Everyone comes as an outpatient, and although many live locally, others are referred by GPs all over the country. Obviously, this kind of service means spending several hours of team members' time with each person, certainly for the initial appointment, so far fewer people can be seen than in a normal hospital outpatient clinic.

The neurorehabilitation unit at the National Hospital for Neurology and Neurosurgery in London is slightly different in that it caters for inpatients who tend to have relatively serious disabilities. However, it is just one part of the neurorehabilitation service offered by the hospital. Initially, people are assessed either on an outpatient or an inpatient basis at the hospital in the centre of London. On the basis of this assessment, individuals may then be offered intensive therapy as an inpatient or an outpatient or they may be referred for treatment locally. The eighteen-bed neurorehabilitation unit is in beautiful grounds in Finchley, north London, and most people usually stay for around 18 to 21 days. While there, they undergo a wide-ranging programme, with the help of a multi-disciplinary team, tailored to their particular needs. The team, led by a consultant neurologist, includes specialist nurses, physiotherapists, speech therapists, occupational therapists and a neuropsychologist and you can also see a social worker, continence advisor and a dietician if you need their advice. The families and carers of people with MS are strongly encouraged to come to the unit and attend assessment meetings and therapy sessions whenever they can.

People who are seen at the main hospital on an outpatient basis will have access to therapists and doctors who have the right expertise to provide whatever treatment or support they need to help them maximize their independence and well-being.

If you are interested in this approach, your neurologist or GP should know whether there is a neurorehabilitation team working anywhere near you, but this may be a problem as the service does not yet cover the whole country. Alternatively, both the National Hospital and the Central Middlesex Neurorehabilitation units are willing to see patients from anywhere, provided they are referred by a doctor.

chapter two

ORTHODOX
MEDICINE

You and your doctors

Once you know you have MS, the kind of relationship you have with your doctors takes on a new importance. If they are supportive and have a good understanding of the condition it can make a big difference as to how well you cope. However, there are many reasons why things don't always work out this way. Relations sometimes start to deteriorate because of delays in diagnosis. Someone who feels they had to battle to convince doctors that their symptoms had a physical rather than a psychological cause may feel bitter and be disinclined to place any trust in the doctors concerned.

The way the doctor gives the news will also have a significant effect and some lack the communication skills to do this sensitively. There's no doubt that some simply feel uncomfortable dealing with a patient whose illness they can't treat effectively or know little about. A GP may have only one patient on his or her list with the condition, and so feel at a bit of a loss as to how to handle them. Some people still find out by accident that they have MS from a junior hospital doctor or other health professional who isn't equipped to deal with the situation. Even when it's the consultant neurologist who gives the diagnosis, he or she may offer little or nothing in the way of information or follow-up. Sometimes you may be told to make another appointment in six months, or you may be given what's called an open-ended appointment – 'Come whenever you feel you need to'. In practice, this often means you never go back at all.

For many people who are newly diagnosed, it's a real shock to discover how little medicine has to offer. A sensitive doctor can lessen the impact by explaining what can be done, as well as what can't. One woman said she felt very encouraged by the neurologist who told her, 'MS may not be curable, but it's certainly helpable!' Sometimes, though, people with MS feel abandoned by the medical profession or that their concerns are not taken seriously. Whether or not this is true in individual cases, it may mean that the person feels justified in directing much of their anger and frustration against their doctors. If the doctors concerned respond to the patient's anger by trying to see as little of them as possible, their future relations are likely to be sterile and unproductive. At this point, a transfer to a different doctor would be a positive move. There may, however, be a temptation to consult a whole succession of doctors in the hope that one will eventually come up with different answers.

Valerie: *'In the early stages I was very ill, and saw one doctor after another in the hope that someone could do something. At one point, I saw that someone had written on my notes "Sees* *far too many doctors" and I realized that was right. Some-times I wanted to break windows and scream at all the doctors because they couldn't do anything – I was so frustrated. Eventually, about ten years ago, I decided to give up doctors – with the exception of my GP – and decided to try and do something for myself. Now I feel much more positive.'*

Chloe: *'I felt when I was given the diagnosis (and still feel) bewildered and a little abandoned by the NHS. By that, I mean the support and information I have received has come from friends, family or as a result of my own research. As this is a disease for which there are few treatments, let alone cures, I feel it would be useful for neurologists to advise on how a patient can manage their own condition, rather than being so dismissive of alternative therapies.'*

If you feel that your relationship with your doctor has disintegrated beyond repair, investigate the possibilities of changing. In principle, changing GPs is simply a question of finding another practice willing to put you on their list and taking along your medical card to register. In reality there may be problems. Popular practices may close their lists to new patients or be unwilling to take on one with long-term health problems. However, if you can find a new practice able to accept you as a patient, they will inform your old doctor and organize the necessary administration. When the problem relates to a hospital doctor, you should be able to get your GP to refer you to someone else, although it may mean transferring to a different hospital.

As you get to know your MS better, you will be the expert on how you are affected by it. You may be someone who is keen to learn as much about the condition as you can, following all the latest research news and finding out as much as possible. Your GP may or may not do the same, but if you are able to build up a good working partnership, you can each benefit from the other's particular knowledge and experience. In many respects, your GP is the 'gatekeeper' to many of the services and treatments you might want or need.

It helps to be clear in your own mind about what you expect from your doctors and to be conscious of the limits to their therapeutic powers. Equally, they have to be able to understand what you want from them – don't expect them to read your mind!

What medicine can offer

Until very recently, doctors had nothing to offer people with MS in the way of treatment that could affect the course of the disease in any way at all. As if the shock of the diagnosis wasn't bad enough, patients had to face up to the fact that not only were there no drugs to cure their condition, there weren't even any which could stop it getting worse.

While it is still true that there is no cure, and no certainty that treatment can arrest the progress of MS, there is at last some light on the horizon. One or two new drugs have been shown in clinical trials to have possible effects on the course of the condition in some people, and research is progressing on others. So far, experts are no more than cautiously optimistic, but that in itself is a considerable step forward. We will look at these new developments in detail in chapter 8, and it is worth talking to your neurologist each time you meet to update yourself on the latest developments.

Meanwhile, efforts may have to be concentrated on

relieving specific symptoms. For many people, the question never arises or does so only occasionally because their symptoms are relatively minor. Nevertheless, it is worth knowing what is available so that you don't miss out on anything which might make your symptoms less troublesome or help you to cope with them better. Even if you manage reasonably well most of the time, you may go through periods when a particular problem gets worse or you have to deal with one that's new to you. Rather than simply struggling on alone, assuming nothing can be done, you should let your doctor know and discuss whether any treatment is available. There may be times when a symptom you associate with your MS actually has some other cause. A need to go to the loo more often than usual, for example, may be a symptom of a urinary infection or cystitis, and it's essential to get the correct medicine to get rid of the problem.

CORTICOSTEROIDS

Many people are reluctant to consider taking this type of drug because they fear that the side effects outweigh any possible benefits. Their sinister reputation stems in part from the fact that they were initially perceived as wonder drugs and over-prescribed before their disadvantages became known. They are also often confused with the related but different anabolic steroids used by some athletes and bodybuilders to increase muscle and strength.

While it is true that they must be used with caution, corticosteroids can often be a big help in relieving symptoms during a relapse and in shortening its duration, especially when inflammation of the optic nerve is causing visual disturbance of some kind. They are thought to work by reducing inflammation which, as we've seen, is the first stage in the destruction of the myelin sheath. They also have an effect on the immune system itself, helping to damp down its abnormal reaction. However, many people who have had steroid treatment say they did not feel any benefit from it. In some cases, it might be that the drugs were not really necessary or appropriate – it has been said that sometimes doctors prescribe them to alleviate their own feelings of helplessness rather than their patients' symptoms!

Be that as it may, used at the right time for the right person, they can be one of the more effective weapons in the MS armoury. Steroids can be given in two ways, intravenously or as tablets, and there are pros and cons to both methods. Intravenous steroids (normally methylprednisolone) are effective, especially for optic neuritis, and have no effect on the gut and fewer side effects generally. Oral treatment (prednisone tablets) can have more noticeable side effects, but there are ways of minimizing the risk of this happening, and oral treatment is not necessarily less effective. Its big advantage over intravenous treatment is that you can have it without going into hospital, which most people would prefer to avoid if possible.

Intravenous therapy is usually given over a period of three to five days, and may sometimes be followed up with a course of tablets. With oral treatment, you start off with a relatively high dose which is then reduced in stages every few days. Studies have shown that steroids are effective in speeding up recovery from acute attacks and used in this way they have no long-term side effects.

It is possible, however, that you will experience some side effects while you are taking them which may take a few days to disappear after the course of treatment has ended. The most noticeable are an increase in appetite, a slight swelling around your face and sometimes a transient growth of facial hair, but these are only temporary changes. Some people experience mood swings or find it difficult to sleep and others complain of having to empty their bladder even more often than usual. The balance of pros and cons will be different for everyone, but despite the problems, many people feel the benefits make it worth putting up with any relatively minor side effects.

However, if steroids are to bring about noticeable improvements, it is important that they are given in the right dose at the right time. Ideally, this should be as close to the start of a relapse or exacerbation as possible and in a large enough dose. Some people find that they are quite effective during a first or second attack, but less so subsequently. A very small minority of people benefit from long-term steroid therapy but this is not appropriate for the majority of people with MS because of problems with unwanted side effects.

Many people with MS have received steroids at some stage, sometimes more than once, with varying results.

Frances: *'I've had intravenous steroids over short periods, and found they really did help me through two very bad relapses.'*

Chloe: *'At one point I lost the use of my right arm and was given a steroid drip daily over a period of three days. It took two to three weeks to begin taking effect, and it's difficult to say with any certainty whether my recovery was actually precipitated by the steroids.'*

William: *'I was given a three-day course of intravenous steroids, and I don't think they helped me. I don't know whether I would have got worse if I didn't have them but I don't seem to have got any better because of them.'*

Janet: *'I have been given steroids on two occasions when I was having very bad attacks, and they helped get me back on my feet.'*

MUSCLE RELAXANTS

Drugs in tablet form such as Baclofen can sometimes make movement easier by releasing spastic muscles. If you have this problem and haven't tried a muscle relaxant before, it could be worth giving it a go. It isn't the answer for everyone because you can end up substituting weakness for the involuntary muscular contraction. Some people find that when their legs are no longer stiff, walking becomes even more difficult than it was before. If this is a problem for you, regular physiotherapy may be a better way to regain some muscular control while avoiding weakness.

Valerie: *'I was prescribed a very low dose of muscle relaxant at my own request because I thought it would help with the muscle pain and seizures. It does help but I only take it when really necessary.'*

Hazel: *'I've been on Baclofen since 1990 and it's good at stopping spasms and allowing my limbs to bend. When I was fifty-five I fell and broke my hip, and have since had a hip replacement operation. I went on a heavy dose immediately afterwards but now it's been cut back down again.'*

ANTIDEPRESSANTS

While virtually everyone who has MS experiences bouts of depression from time to time, not everyone needs treatment with antidepressant medicines. They can't do anything about the cause of your gloom in so far as it is triggered by the effect your condition has on your life, but recent evidence suggests that they may have a positive effect on depression which arises from the neurological changes MS brings about. Specifically, plaques or lesions on certain parts of the brain can directly affect your emotional responses and control.

In the long term, of course, there is no alternative to evolving your own solution to the problems of living with MS – a process which is likely to be ongoing. You may need to talk to others who have shared similar experiences, to your family and friends, to professional counsellors or spiritual advisors.

In the meantime, antidepressants can be helpful if depression gets such a grip on you that making any effort seems quite beyond you. It is important that you (or someone close to you) should seek the necessary help from your GP in such a situation. Sadly, many people still believe that a depressed person should be able to snap out of it and pull themselves together, but you can no more do that than you could snap out of a broken leg or flu. A course of antidepressants can lift your mood sufficiently to enable you to benefit from 'talking therapies' or to begin working through your own feelings about your MS. Modern drugs have few if any side effects and you cannot become dependent on them so there is no risk of withdrawal symptoms when you stop taking them.

Don't be shocked if your doctor suggests an antidepressant when you feel you are coping well psychologically. In addition to their main role in lifting depression, this type of drug is sometimes helpful in easing certain kinds of pain associated with MS, especially burning sensations in your hands and feet.

William: *'I became very depressed after I had been diagnosed, and was sent to a private clinic by my firm. They referred me to a psychiatrist who prescribed antidepressants and a course of counselling, which were very helpful.'*

PAIN RELIEF

Help may be available for certain kinds of pain and the form it takes will depend on exactly what kind of pain you're experiencing.

- **Trigeminal neuralgia**. This is caused by inflammation of the base of the trigeminal nerve which supplies the nerves in your face and the stabbing pains are worse than toothache. Fortunately, many people find it can be relieved or at least eased by a drug called carbamazepine.
- **Muscular pain**. You may be putting undue stresses on various parts of your musculo-skeletal system by the way you sit, stand or move. A properly designed chair (or a better wheelchair) which gives support to your lower back, plus help from a physiotherapist to improve your gait and strengthen the muscles in your lower back may alleviate these types of aches and pains.

Treating bladder problems

For most of us, difficulties of this kind are one of the last unmentionables, a subject we're reluctant to broach even with our nearest and dearest. This reticence means people are less likely to be aware of the various means available of tackling the problem or to ask for information and help when they need it. In fact, continence problems are extremely common, affecting around 70 per cent of people with MS at some point and many other people besides.

There are a number of ways in which bladder control can go wrong as a result of MS and a variety of approaches to overcoming any particular problem. You may find that you can solve yours for yourself with a bit of thought and advance planning, but sometimes it can be more complicated. Your doctor may be able to offer some help by way of medical treatment, depending on the nature and severity of your problem.

- **What goes wrong**. Normal bladder control can be disrupted either by changes to the bladder muscle itself and/or the sphincter muscle which controls the outflow of urine or by myelin damage to the nerves responsible for maintaining communications between bladder and brain.
- **What treatment is available**. When your bladder becomes overactive, forcing you to hurry to the loo very frequently, you may find that drugs (called anticholinergics) help by relaxing the bladder muscle so that it can stretch to hold more urine. There are other drugs which can help with the opposite problem – when the bladder seems reluctant to empty or does so incompletely. Alternatively, you may be able to use a catheter – a fine tube passed into the bladder when you need to empty it. This procedure is called 'intermittent self-catheterization' and is the approach most commonly used today. It's possible to have a catheter which remains permanently in place, but this is done relatively rarely nowadays. Other aids, such as incontinence pads, are also

among the options, which need to be tailored to your personal requirements, usually with the help of a specialist continence advisor (see page 158). Sometimes, antibiotics may be suggested as a precaution against urinary infections which are more likely when the bladder doesn't empty completely.

Common sense might seem to suggest that it's a good idea to cut down on the amount of liquids you drink to reduce the need to go to the loo frequently. However, this isn't a good idea as you may end up taking too little fluid. Similarly, emptying your bladder (or trying to) more and more often 'just in case' isn't as useful a ploy as it sounds because it may just train your bladder to hold a smaller amount of urine before demanding to be emptied.

For many people, symptoms involving the bladder come and go, but for those with a long-term problem there are further options available. In such cases, arriving at a solution that's right for each individual is likely to be a team effort, involving you and possibly your doctor, a physiotherapist, district (or community) nurse and a specialist continence advisor. We will consider these options in chapter 8.

Treating bowel problems

Complete loss of bowel control is relatively rare in MS, but damage to nerve pathways can lead to muscle weakness and can make bowel emptying difficult. Sometimes, people may lose the sensation which tells them that their bowel needs emptying. It is usually possible, with the help of your GP and/or a specialist continence advisor, to manage the problem with reasonable effectiveness, even when control is lost completely. As with bladder problems, difficulties with bowel control need to be managed on an individual basis. Bowel problems are often improved if you can avoid becoming constipated as this can lead to overflow diarrhoea. Including more fibre in your diet is very important, so try to eat as much fresh vegetables and fruit as possible, plus cereals and opt for wholemeal bread, rice and pasta rather than white. If you would like specific guidance on making changes, ask your doctor to refer you to a dietician. A continence advisor may also suggest ways to help the situation such as getting into a regular routine of opening your bowels and possibly taking gentle exercise to stimulate the bowel.

Eye problems

Eye pain and reduced vision – optic neuritis – is often one of the first symptoms of MS and usually disappears in time. Sometimes, steroid treatment can help speed up the recovery, and it can also be useful if you suffer double vision during a relapse. People who experience the flickering of the eyes known as nystagmus can sometimes be treated with drugs, including injecting a muscle relaxant called botulinum into the muscles of the eye.

Fatigue

Most people with MS suffer from this problem, and when you do, you will almost certainly have to make adjustments to your lifestyle to allow for it. However, various treatments have been tried, and a drug called Amantadine has proved beneficial for some people with MS fatigue.

Vitamin B12

Weekly or monthly injections are sometimes given to people with MS by their GPs. Although many people say they feel better as a result, there is no medical evidence that they do any measurable good. However, there have been reports suggesting that some people with MS may have lower than normal levels of B12, so some would argue that they might benefit from having injections.

The treatment was originally devised for people suffering from pernicious anaemia, who experienced neurological symptoms due to a gut problem which prevented them absorbing vitamin B12 from their diet. The theory was that if it helped with neurological symptoms, then people with MS might benefit from the same treatment. Unfortunately, there is a fault in this logic: the majority of people with MS are quite capable of absorbing all the vitamin B12 they need from their diet and their neurological symptoms are therefore not caused by any deficiency. Nevertheless, doctors who have little else by way of treatment to offer to people with MS are sometimes willing to prescribe it on the grounds that it does no harm and allows both parties to feel that something positive is being done.

Physiotherapy

In an ideal world, most people with MS could probably benefit from regular, frequent sessions with a physiotherapist with special knowledge of their condition. A personalized programme of selected exercises, adapted to take account of any new or worsening symptoms, can help to minimize the effects of muscle stiffness and poor coordination, maintain muscle tone and improve balance. Many people have found that regular physiotherapy has improved their mobility and balance in particular, relaxed spastic muscles and given them better control over their arms and hands. If it is started at a relatively early stage, it can also prevent you developing bad posture habits to compensate for any difficulties in sitting, standing and walking.

Of course, in this ideal world, the person with MS would continue to practise the exercise programme at home, even when they were relatively symptom-free, but without pushing themselves too hard! In practice, of course, most people are tempted to backslide when things are going well, and in any case getting access to the right amount and type of physiotherapy on the NHS is not always easy or even possible.

Physiotherapists mostly work in hospitals, but there are

some who are based in the community and able to visit patients in their own homes. Obviously, this can have particular advantages for someone who has mobility problems or who experiences a lot of fatigue. Often just getting to the hospital, even if transport is provided, involves so much effort that you're not fit for anything by the time you arrive. Some local authority day centres also offer physiotherapy, and could be easier to get to.

Whether you are following an exercise programme at a physiotherapy unit or at home, it is essential that you find the right balance between doing too little and too much. Of course, this may well be different for you at different times and it's counterproductive to press on regardless when your symptoms indicate that a rest is in order. You will simply end up exhausted which does you no good at all. However, it is possible to continue with physiotherapy even at times when your voluntary movement is restricted: the physio can gently manipulate your limbs to release contracted muscles and it should help you to regain their use more easily when the acute phase has passed. Some hospitals have special pools for patients receiving physiotherapy, and some people find them beneficial or at least enjoy using them. Usually the water is heated to a higher temperature than a normal swimming pool, however, and many people with MS find the fatigue brought on by the warmth counteracts any benefits from the exercise itself. The only way to find out if it affects you in this way is to try it if the option is there and the idea appeals.

Referral to an NHS physiotherapy unit is through your neurologist or GP and, depending on the availability of the service in your area, you may have to make do with fewer sessions than you would like. It is possible to go privately if you can afford it, but do ask either your GP or neurologist for a recommendation before choosing a practitioner.

Alternatively, group sessions led by a neurologically trained physiotherapist are available at many local MS centres; contact the the MS Resource Centre (address on page 201) for a list.

> **Janet:** *'I was referred to a physiotherapist immediately after I'd been given the diagnosis – I think it was partly that my neurologist was desperate to be able to offer me something, and that was all there was! In fact, I found it was very helpful at first, and I carried on doing exercises at a local hospital gym and at home when I couldn't get there. It seemed to be especially good at maintaining my strength, but recently my symptoms have got worse, especially fatigue, and I just haven't had the energy for it. I probably ought to give it another try because it was good.'*

3 COMPLEMENTARY THERAPIES

There are many reasons why people turn to complementary medicine and, to some extent, what you get out of it may depend on your expectations. The first thing that has to be said is that, like their colleagues in orthodox medicine, no therapist is in a position to promise a cure for your MS. In fact, very few are likely to do so, but you'd be wise to be wary of anyone who even hinted at the possibility. From time to time, new 'treatments' appear whose proponents claim remarkable effects on the symptoms of those with MS who've followed them. There are usually plenty of people who report that their symptoms disappeared once they started on the regime, whatever it may be, and naturally they assume that these two facts are cause and effect. It is tempting to give such treatments a try in the hope that you too will benefit to the same degree, but so far, no direct link has been proven between any of these approaches and the disappearance of MS symptoms. However, since the same is largely true of orthodox medicine, you may still decide to go ahead on the grounds that you've nothing to lose and everything to gain.

While many members of the medical profession are

becoming more open-minded about complementary medicine, you are still likely to get a cautious if not discouraging reaction when you raise the subject. Doctors are trained to think scientifically and so are likely to point out that there is no evidence that any of these therapies can affect the course of MS. While this is true, they may have more subtle benefits, not the least of which is the time and concern for you as an individual which most therapists offer. Any treatment which you feel has a beneficial effect on you is worthwhile, whether it actually alleviates your symptoms, helps to boost your general health or gives you a psychological lift. In addition, many people with MS say that simply doing something positive reduces their sense of frustration and helplessness: at least they're taking back some degree of control rather than just waiting passively for the medics to come up with answers. Nevertheless, doctors and others involved professionally in the care of people with MS worry that complementary therapy may offer false hope which can only lead ultimately to disappointment, leaving you worse off than before. Obviously this can and does happen with some people, but the majority are not that naive.

If you do want to consider some form of complementary medicine, there are a few points you should consider before you embark on it.

- With the exception of osteopathy and chiropractic, anyone can set themselves up as a therapist without any checks being made on their training, experience or competence. Refer to one of the reputable organizations (see pages 206–9) before choosing your therapist. Members will have had some kind of training and although registration is no guarantee of quality, it is at least a starting point.

- Ask questions of your chosen therapist: what does treatment involve, what does it cost, how long does each session last and how many will you need before expecting to feel some benefit? Do you have to go to them, or can they do the treatment in your own home?
- It's probably best to undergo one treatment at a time. That way, you will be better able to assess whether a particular therapy is doing you any good. If you have several simultaneously, you won't be able to tell which, if any, is worthwhile. What's more, having several sessions with different practitioners each week can leave you exhausted and confused by the clash of philosophies.
- Try to clarify in your own mind how you will measure success. You may decide that if a particular treatment makes you feel more relaxed, more positive or less helpless then it's worth your time and money. You may feel that the benefits are more psychological than physical, but that could give you reason enough to continue. On the other hand, if you're looking for an improvement in your symptoms which isn't forthcoming, you may want to give up on that particular therapy. Some people like to set a limit in advance: I'll stop if I don't feel any benefit after x sessions. Otherwise, you may end up like some of those who go for psychoanalysis, seeing your therapist for years on end in the hope that improvement is just around the corner and spending a small fortune in the meantime!

Acupuncture

This ancient system of Chinese medicine aims to promote good health by adjusting the balance between two opposing forces – Yin and Yang. Yin is passive and is represented by water, while Yang is active and is represented by fire. Therapists use traditional acupuncture points which lie along the 'meridians' or energy pathways which are believed to conduct vital energy (Ki) through your body. By stimulating the appropriate points with very fine needles, the acupuncturist fine tunes the energy flow to right the balance between Yin and Yang. The needles aren't painful, although you may feel a dull ache for a few seconds as they penetrate the skin through to the acupuncture point. The needles may be left in place for a few moments or up to an hour, and sometimes a mild electric current may be transmitted to them, giving you a slight tingling feeling.

Which of the possible points are chosen and how long the needles are left in will be decided on the basis of a detailed discussion with the acupuncturist about your symptoms, life history, state of mind and so on. You will probably also be given a physical examination.

While some people say that they feel better after just one or two sessions of acupuncture, others may need a number of treatments and some will find it makes no difference to them at all.

In recent years, Western doctors who have investigated acupuncture have suggested alternative explanations as to why it may be effective. One of the more popular theories is that the needle stimulation triggers the release of chemicals called endorphins, which are sometimes referred to as the body's natural painkillers. As far as some orthodox medical practitioners are concerned, acupuncture is one of the more 'respectable' complementary therapies and some GPs even provide it in their surgeries! If yours doesn't, you can get a list of practitioners from one of the organizations listed on pages 206–9.

> **Valerie:** *'I still have acupuncture sometimes when I feel I need re-energizing, and at one time I had quite a lot of sessions. I liked it because it made me feel physically lighter as well as leaving me with much more energy.'*

Acupressure and Shiatsu

These are based on the same principles as acupuncture, but without the use of needles. Shiatsu is the Japanese form, and although the word literally means 'finger pressure', the therapist may also apply pressure using the palms of the hands, or even the elbows, feet and knees. It's sometimes said to be a combination of acupuncture and massage and many people learn it to use as a form of home remedy or first aid. However, as a person with MS, you should only consult a practitioner who has studied the art in depth; contact the Shiatsu Society, address on page 209.

Aromatherapy

The word literally means 'treatment with scents', which may involve massage, baths, creams, compresses and vapours. Essential oils, extracted from plants, flowers and other natural sources are, with a very few exceptions, always used in a diluted form. For massage, a few drops are added to a carrier oil, or the oils may be mixed with water for other uses such as in a bath or for inhalation. They are said to achieve their effects by two means: through the smell which you breathe in and by absorption through the skin.

The therapist will discuss your personal situation and symptoms, then select and combine particular oils according to their individual properties to meet your particular needs. For example, rosemary may be chosen if you have neuro-muscular problems, or juniper oil, which has diuretic properties, for water retention.

An aromatherapy massage is an enjoyable and relaxing experience, and many people with MS find it helps, especially with stress and fatigue. Even if you don't want to consult an aromatherapist, you may like to try using the oils at home. As well as toiletries, you can also buy candles and other products which scent the air. Remember that essential oils shouldn't be used undiluted on your skin, but many of the commercially available ones come already mixed with carrier oils.

Aromatherapy is another complementary therapy which is now being offered as an adjunct to conventional treatment in some hospitals and doctors' surgeries. You can get information about local practitioners from the International Federation of Aromatherapists, address on page 208.

Chloe: *'I like using essential oils in my bath and sometimes on my pillow at night. I find lavender and geranium are good for me.'*

Frances: *'I find that regular aromatherapy massage really does help to reduce tension – the problem for me is that it's expensive!'*

Healing

The actual techniques used by healers and their underlying philosophies vary widely, but all feel they have the gift of helping others who are sick in body or mind. It is rare to find one who will offer a miracle cure or even any guarantee of improvement and it is irrelevant whether you happen to share their particular belief system. They may personally believe that their gift comes from God or that it is inspired by a spiritual guide, but their shared aim is to channel the healing gift to the people they treat. Often, this is done by the so-called 'laying on of hands' or sometimes with the healer's hands held close to the patient's body. Many people who have been treated in this way say they feel a definite sensation – often of heat – during the healing session and an immediate easing of their symptoms, while others says the benefits are mainly psychological. And, of course, some find it has no effect on them at all.

Most healers are ordinary people who feel they have somehow been given this gift and are anxious simply to use it to help others. It is not uncommon for healers to offer their services free or in return for a voluntary donation, although many full-time healers do charge, but the cost is usually reasonable. While there are many convincing stories of people who are certain that healing has worked for them, no one can say what, if anything, is really happening. It may be all in the mind or it may be some as yet unrecognized but real power, but provided you don't go expecting miracles, it's likely to do more good than harm. To contact a reputable healer in your area, write to the National Federation of Spiritual Healers, address on page 208.

Jenny: *'A cousin suggested taking me to see a healer who she knew and although I wasn't expecting much I agreed to go. She was a very warm, sympathetic woman and didn't make any promises that she could help my MS. When she held her hands over me, I felt a definite sensation of warmth, and afterwards my legs seemed to be less stiff for a short time. I saw her a second time with the same result. I can't say my symptoms improved, but I found it a worthwhile experience, and there was no charge, although I did make a voluntary donation.'*

Herbal remedies

Herbal medicine (or phytotherapy) has been in use throughout human history, although it's only relatively recently that scientists have begun analysing and identifying the active components of many traditional remedies. Today, medical herbalists still use a combination of herbal preparations and changes to patients' diets when appropriate. As with all complementary therapies, treatment will be decided on the basis of a detailed personal history with reference to your particular symptoms. It may well include a herb called St John's wort which is considered to have a beneficial effect on the nervous system. It is sometimes used in combination with a special tonic prepared from oats which is thought to stimulate and improve nerve function.

Some people assume that because herbalism uses only natural herbs and foods, it is quite safe, but some of the constituents can have powerful effects and it's important to get expert advice before treating yourself. You can find out more and get a list of registered practitioners from The National Institute of Medical Herbalists, address on page 209.

Homoeopathy

This is based on principles set out in the eighteenth century by the German physician Dr Samuel Hahnemann and concentrates on treating the whole person rather than a specific disease or symptom. In fact, two people with apparently identical symptoms would be unlikely to be prescribed the same homoeopathic remedies because other factors about the individual concerned would also be taken into account.

There is an enormous number of possible remedies prepared from plants, minerals and other sources which may be used singly or in combination. The fundamental idea behind homoeopathy is that 'like cures like': in other words, the chosen remedy will be one which would be expected to produce the symptoms you are experiencing. Most homoeopathic remedies come in the form of small, lactose-based pills to which have been added a few drops of solution prepared from the original substance. The process of preparation involves many stages of dilution, to the point where it is impossible to detect any trace of the original substance. Just how the remedies achieve their effect is not clear, even to homoeopaths, and leads many people to question whether they can possibly work at all.

When you consult a homoeopath, you will be asked a lot of questions to enable the therapist to choose the appropriate treatment, which will be designed to encourage your body's powers of self-healing. Although you may initially experience a worsening of symptoms, this is said to be a sign of the treatment's effectiveness. There are no side effects and the remedies are entirely safe.

Homoeopathy is the only complementary therapy which has long been part of the NHS, since 1948 in fact, and there are many doctors – both in hospitals and general practice – who are also qualified homoeopaths. In theory, you should be able to get treatment through the NHS, but in practice this will depend on local policy in your area. There are also many lay homoeopaths practising privately and you can get a list of those in your area from the British Homoeopathic Association, address on page 207.

Lizzy: *'I had treatment at the Royal London Homoeopathic Hospital on the NHS shortly after getting my diagnosis. Originally I was taking Nat Mur which did seem to help my bladder problems at first but then stopped working. I've also taken Causticum and I find Kali Phos very good for my insomnia.'*

Hyperbaric oxygen (HBO)

What this treatment actually entails is breathing high pressure (hyperbaric) oxygen through a face mask while sitting in a metal chamber something like a diving bell in a controlled atmosphere. It is important that this is done in properly controlled and supervised conditions or it could be dangerous. Before considering it, you should check with your GP to make sure there are no specific reasons why you should avoid pressurization, such as acute sinus trouble or ear or chest problems.

When it was first popularized in the early 1980s, HBO was claimed as a real breakthrough in the treatment of MS, but subsequent research has not justified the original excitement. The theory is that breathing pressurized oxygen can slow or even stop the inflammation of the myelin sheath which is the precursor of plaque formation, but there is no evidence that this actually occurs. Nevertheless, some people with MS continue to have weekly HBO sessions and say that they feel less fatigued and more energetic and sometimes that they have fewer bladder problems after what they often call 'a dive'.

For information about where to try HBO, contact one of the MS therapy centres or the MS Resource Centre, addresses on pages 201–2.

Hypnotherapy

Hypnosis is now one of the approaches offered at specialist pain clinics and is also used to help people recognize and relieve stresses and tension. Therapists may use the technique as a means of enabling you to express your hidden fears and emotions as well as offering strategies to deal with pain. Some people feel uncomfortable at the prospect of being hypnotized, but you need have no fear that you will be made to do anything embarrassing or to behave in ways that would be unacceptable to you normally.

For more information, contact The British Society of Medical and Dental Hypnosis, telephone number on page 207.

Massage

Massage can be a great way to ease tension and promote a feeling of well-being and relaxation. It can take several sessions before you really feel the benefit, and it may be better to have relatively short sessions while you're getting used to the experience. If the person giving the massage doesn't know very much about MS, you should explain the basics and what symptoms you have.

Most people feel tired after a massage, so it's best avoided when you're suffering from fatigue. It can also provoke muscular spasms if you aren't very relaxed, so may not help if that is one of your major symptoms. Stick to the same masseur if you find you enjoy the treatment and they will get to know what suits you best.

For more information, contact the London College of Massage, address on page 208.

Osteopathy and chiropractic

These are both forms of manipulative therapy, though using different techniques, and some people with MS have found them helpful in resolving postural problems. You would need to find a practitioner who understands your condition and a relatively small number of sessions should be enough to indicate whether the treatment is beneficial for you. Ask your GP for a referral or contact one of the organizations mentioned on page 207.

Reflexology

The underlying principle of reflexology is that the structure of your whole body is mirrored in your feet – almost like a miniaturized relief map. Reflexologists believe that the body can be divided into ten energy zones – five on each side – and that every part of your anatomy has its counterpart in a reflex point on your feet. This is why reflexology is also sometimes known as zone therapy.

At your first meeting, the therapist will spend time going into your medical history and getting to know you as a person. The actual treatment consists of massage to specific areas of the feet, determined by your particular needs and symptoms.

No one is really sure how reflexology works, but at the very least, it should leave you feeling relaxed and with an overall sense of well-being. At best, you may find that pain and stiffness are eased, at least for a while, and that you have greater mobility and energy. Initially, treatment is weekly, usually around six to eight sessions, but many people choose to continue beyond that, either on a regular basis or now and again. Many reflexologists are happy to come to your home, which is an extra plus point if your mobility is limited.

For more information, contact the International Federation of Reflexology, address on page 208.

Yoga

Yoga is not a form of complementary therapy, but the many people with MS who practise it do so because they find it has positive health benefits. Based on an ancient eastern philosophy and system of controlled breathing and movement, it is a way of taking control of your mind and body and bringing them into harmony. Beginners will usually learn specific breathing techniques to start with, and one of the advantages of yoga is that many of the postures and movements can be performed by, or adapted for, those who are not fully physically fit.

Many people with MS make a point of finding time for their daily sessions because they say yoga helps relieve stress and maximize energy, as well as toning up muscles and keeping the body supple. Enthusiasts point out that it's worth keeping at it for a while if you find the techniques difficult or the approach a little off-putting at first. The aim is to harness your personal energy and potential to help you take charge of your life in a holistic and non-competitive way which well repays the effort involved in mastering the techniques.

Many teachers run classes which allow for the individual needs of people with MS, and you can get details of those in your area from The Yoga for Health Foundation, which runs a residential centre as well as local groups around the country (address on page 209).

Chloe: *'I go to yoga once a week which I find useful as it alleviates stress and puts me in tune with my body. I have a tendency to live in spite of my body rather than with it, and yoga is teaching me to be comfortable with it and be aware of its strengths as well as its limitations.'*

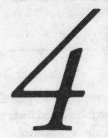

chapter four

SELF-HELP APPROACHES TO TREATMENT

F rom time to time, you'll probably hear about lifestyle changes or particular remedies which have been tried with greater or lesser success by other people with MS. The decision as to whether the costs, inconvenience or practical difficulties of each approach are justified by the possible benefits is one only you can make. As with the complementary therapies, none has, as yet, been proven to have any effect on the neurological changes underlying MS. Nevertheless, all have their advocates who are convinced that the benefits for them are real. It's worth bearing in mind that some may involve a considerable financial outlay, and you may like to consider setting yourself a limit as to how much money and time you are prepared to devote to them to see whether they work for you.

Dietary changes

A HEALTHY EATING PLAN

There is no doubt that all of us have something to gain healthwise from eating the right kind of well-balanced diet, whether or not we have MS. In addition, there is evidence that adjusting the balance of fats in your diet so you get more of the so-called essential fatty acids may reduce the severity – and possibly the frequency – of relapses for people with MS.

Adopting a healthy diet means choosing foods that will provide sufficient (but not too many) calories and all the nutrients your body needs to maintain itself. For most of us, it also means cutting down on foods which provide few nutritional benefits and which may have an adverse effect on our overall health. It is worth asking your doctor to refer you to a dietician if you are confused about what you should be eating or need advice about how to change your diet. However, the basic guidelines are relatively straightforward:

- **Reduce your overall fat intake**. In particular, you should eat less saturated fat – which mostly comes from animal sources and is usually hard at room temperature. As well as the obvious things like fatty meat and butter, you need to watch out for the fat content of prepared foods such as pies, full-fat dairy products, sausages and so on. Whenever possible, opt for unsaturated fats which are found mostly in vegetable oils (with the exception of coconut and palm oil) and some fish oils.

Research studies have indicated that MS appears to be more prevalent in parts of the world where people normally eat more saturated fats, and thus less of the unsaturated kind.

In addition, people with MS were found to have lower than normal levels of polyunsaturated fats in their bloodstream, possibly because their bodies' processing mechanisms were defective. These findings are important because the so-called essential polyunsaturated fatty acids are converted by the body into other acids with slightly different chemical structures and used in the brain and nervous system for repair and maintenance. They therefore maintain the myelin sheath and also play a role in the efficient operation of the immune system. The main essential fatty acids are linoleic, linolenic and arachnidonic acids, all of which can be derived from certain foods. Following the studies on the relationship between MS and unsaturated fats, trials designed to assess the effect of linoleic acid supplements on the course of the condition showed that people taking them had fewer severe relapses than a control group who were taking dummy capsules, and that their relapses did not last as long. The capsules used in the trials were sunflower seed oil, but linoleic acid can also be taken in capsules based on other oils, including safflower, corn, soya, rapeseed and oil of evening primrose. They are not available on prescription, but although you can buy them from health food shops, taking them on a long-term basis can cost a fair bit. In any case, you can achieve the same effect by taking polyunsaturated fats in their natural form in your normal diet.

Chloe: *'I take evening primrose oil – twelve capsules a day – which I find useful. When I had my first major relapse, I had stopped taking it for about six months and since then I've been taking it again. It seems to have helped, but it's difficult to say with any certainty.'*

- **Eat the right kind of carbohydrates**. This means cutting down on 'simple' carbohydrates – sugars – in particular refined sugar and foods sweetened with it. At the same time, you should also try to increase your consumption of complex carbohydrates (or fibre) which are found in foods such as cereals, fruit, vegetables, seeds and pulses. It can take a while to get used to the different texture of high fibre versions of familiar foods, such as wholemeal pasta, brown rice or wholemeal bread and, in any case, upping your fibre intake too suddenly can be a shock to your digestive system. You're less likely to suffer from stomachache or wind if you make the change gradually and that will also give you time to re-educate your tastebuds if you have a naturally sweet tooth.

- **Don't worry about protein**. Although it is essential for body repair and maintenance, you are virtually certain to be getting enough to meet your needs. Nutritionists suggest that we would all do better to increase the proportion of vegetable protein in our diets at the expense of the kind derived from animal sources. This means eating more nuts, pulses, vegetables, fruit and bread, and less meat, dairy produce and eggs.

- **Vitamins and minerals**. A varied diet containing plenty of fresh food should usually supply all your body's requirements without the need for supplements. Vitamins and minerals consumed in their natural form – in food – are, in any case, thought to do more good than artificially extracted ones. However, if your diet is restricted for some reason, if your appetite is poor or if you have problems with chewing, swallowing or digestion, you might benefit from boosting your intake of certain vitamins or minerals. It would be worth discussing the situation with your GP or a dietician if you think this could apply to you. Injections of vitamin B12 are sometimes given as a treatment for MS but there is no evidence that it is effective for the majority of people (see page 52).

There are a number of sources of information and inspiration which you may find useful if you're planning to switch to a healthier diet. *Enjoy Good Food,* published by the MS Society, has interesting background information plus a selection of recipes, and is available from the address on page 201. *Eating and MS,* published by the Multiple Sclerosis Resource Centre, has lots of recipes to help you follow a healthy eating plan including foods rich in essential fatty acids. It is available from the MSRC, address on page 201.

You do need to be careful about putting on too much extra weight. This can make mobility problems worse and have other undesirable effects on your health. Unfortunately, this can be something of a problem, especially if your MS prevents you from being as active as you once were or makes sport or exercise virtually impossible. There's also the temptation to nibble out of boredom or for comfort if your MS has restricted your lifestyle. Ask to see a dietician if you would like advice on keeping your weight down. You can also get a leaflet on '*Slimming tips*' from the MS Resource Centre, address on page 201.

Alcohol

Drinking in moderation is not thought to do anyone any harm and there have even been recent reports of possible health benefits from drinking a small amount regularly every day – say two small glasses of wine, a single measure of spirits or a pint of beer. However, there are a few extra considerations to take into account when you have MS. For one thing, you can take in quite a lot of extra calories which will fuel any tendency to gain unwanted weight. For another, some of the physical effects produced by drinking alcohol are similar to some of the possible symptoms of MS – poor coordination, lack of balance and impaired concentration, for example. In this situation, you may feel the effects of drinking rather more rapidly than you might have done previously.

A few people may be tempted to drown their sorrows in alcohol but this inevitably generates more problems than it solves. Overindulgence will have health consequences for someone with MS just as it would for anyone, but ordinary social drinking will have no impact on the course of your condition.

Sue: *'On a frivolous note, I find that I become legless very quickly these days – so I always sit down before drinking. After all, everyone should be encouraged to drink safely.'*

Gluten-free diet

In recent years, some people with MS have avoided eating any food containing gluten – found in wheat and foods made from it – in the belief that this was the way to put their symptoms into remission. Much of the enthusiasm stemmed from a booklet written by Robert McDougall, who is convinced that his long remission is due to the diet he devised for himself in the late 1960s. As well as cutting out all foods containing gluten, he also stopped eating milk products and refined sugar, making up for any resulting vitamin and mineral deficiencies by taking supplements. The story of his apparent recovery is certainly dramatic, but the problem is that there is no evidence that a similar diet would have the same effect on anyone else.

Following a gluten-free diet is not particularly easy. Apart from the fact that you can't have ordinary bread, pasta, pastry, cakes or biscuits, you also have to study the small print of all food labelling and question staff in restaurants and takeaways closely to determine whether any trace of wheat products such as flour might be present in anything you're thinking of eating. It involves a lot of effort and self-denial which is unlikely to bring any tangible reward to make it worthwhile.

Cannabis

Both in this country and elsewhere, people with MS have found that cannabis has relieved some of their symptoms when nothing else had any effect whatsoever. It is said by many of them to be particularly effective in relieving muscle spasm, tremor, pain, loss of balance and bladder problems. They feel that it is more effective than conventional muscle-relaxant drugs and has fewer unpleasant side effects.

There have been relatively few clinical studies of its effectiveness, but those which have been conducted tend to support the claims made by people with MS who have tried it for themselves. According to a survey carried out among hospital doctors in 1994 by the magazine *BMA News Review*, many believe that cannabis should be available on prescription for the relatively small number of people whose symptoms justify its use. In fact, it was possible to obtain it in this way until 1971, when the law was changed because of the risk of misuse.

Currently there are two main problems in using the drug. First, the cultivation, possession and use of cannabis are illegal, even for symptom relief rather than for recreation. Secondly, many people find that the most effective way to take cannabis is in cigarettes, and this carries all the health risks associated with ordinary smoking. Some people get round this by crumbling small amounts into food – usually home-made biscuits – then cooking it, or alternatively brewing a kind of tea using the dried leaves. However, this does not take effect as quickly as smoking it mixed with tobacco or dried herbs. It's also easier to tell how much you're taking when you smoke it. The average medicinal dose is a pea-sized portion of resin per day, which in most cases is unlikely to be enough to produce the mood change which is the goal of recreational users.

Obviously, because cannabis is illegal, everyone must make their own decision as to whether they want to try it. Those who do normally ask around friends or family – and are often surprised at how easy it is to get hold of, even through their most respectable acquaintances!

If you prefer not to to try it while it is illegal – or even if that doesn't especially worry you – you might like to join ACT, the Alliance for Cannabis Therapeutics. Described by its founder Clare Hodges, who has MS herself, as 'a Patients' Organization', ACT campaigns to have cannabis made available on prescription for those who could benefit medically from its use. A delegation comprising members plus sympathetic doctors and politicians has already outlined their case to the Department of Health, who have promised to consider the possibility of changing the legal position. For more information about the organization and its work, send four first class stamps, with your name and address, to ACT, PO Box CR14, Leeds LS7 4XF.

Clare: *'I've had MS for fourteen years, and one of my symptoms has been bladder problems. I've used self-catheterization to empty my bladder, which is no big deal, but my bladder muscle was in constant spasm, which made me feel as if I was always bursting to go to the loo, even when I knew I didn't need to. I'd had endless drugs, including muscle relaxants, but nothing had been any use at all. The problem got so bad I hardly slept at night, which made all my day-time symptoms worse – I could hardly see or walk. Then a friend who has MS told me about reports in American medical journals which discussed using cannabis to relieve symptoms both in MS and some other conditions.*

When I tried it, I found it relieved my symptoms in a way nothing else had. As well as easing the bladder problem, it stopped the spasms in my spine which were very uncomfortable. Unlike the muscle-relaxant drugs, it allowed me to maintain motor control while taking away the spasms. I feel very strongly that people who could benefit from taking cannabis for medical reasons should be able to get it on prescription, and preferably in a form which didn't involve smoking.'

Cari Loder

Since appearing on TV and the publication of her autobiography *Standing in the Sunshine* in 1996, Cari Loder has received a great deal of media coverage. She began following a combined treatment regime of her own devising in 1994, and her MS symptoms have gone into total remission. Cari is positive that the improvement in her health is a result of the treatment, although she does not claim to be cured of MS.

She had been diagnosed two years previously as having primary progressive MS and her condition had been deteriorating without any periods of remission. Within that time, she had developed very severe disabilities which had brought her to the point of considering suicide. Reluctantly, she allowed her GP to prescribe a course of antidepressants. Her symptoms began to improve within ten days, and gradually disappeared entirely.

Her analysis of what happened is that a chance combination of these antidepressants with vitamin B12 injections and an amino acid derived from drinking masses of diet cola was the direct cause of this dramatic improvement. Although the precise recipe for her treatment cocktail was initially passed on to other people with MS, this has now stopped in preparation for a clinical trial planned to start in early 1997. According to Cari, it is essential to combine exactly the right ingredients made by the same manufacturers as those she herself used, so DIY guesses are pointless.

The trial is expected to last for around eighteen months and the results will have to be analysed, so no further information is likely to appear for some time. In the meantime, it has to be said that doctors are sceptical to put it very mildly. They can see no reason why such a combination of ingredients should have any effect on MS symptoms, and are also concerned about possible side effects such as increased pulse rate and raised blood pressure in some people.

5

DIGESTING THE NEWS

The new reality

No one can know what it feels like to discover that you have
MS unless they have been through it themselves. Even when
they have, their reaction is bound to differ to some degree
from yours because you are a unique individual. You may
well find that you share some of the same feelings and
worries, but much will depend on your circumstances, on
your personality, on the severity of your illness and its
nature, and on your relationships with other people. What
almost everyone can agree on, however, is that something
fundamental has changed. Life will never be quite the same
again, even if you are one of those whose symptoms remain
relatively trivial or who experience very long periods of
remission. Ultimately, of course, each person has to find
their own way of living with the reality of their MS, but that
doesn't mean you have to do it on your own. Information,
advice and support are on offer from a variety of sources,
including many people who have faced and are facing some
of the same difficulties. In this chapter and the next we'll be

looking at some of the emotional and psychological aspects of MS as they affect both people with the condition and others involved with them. Not all will be relevant to you personally but if you can identify with some of the situations discussed, you may find it helpful to know how others have dealt with them.

FINDING OUT

Your immediate reaction to the diagnosis of MS may be coloured by what you were expecting. Many people say they were not actually surprised, while for others the news came out of a clear blue sky. Sometimes, there's even an element of relief – at last you know what's been causing those weird symptoms. Neither you nor anyone else can now put them down to hypochondria or neurosis. For a minority, the news may actually be better than what they had feared.

> **Jenny**: *'When my GP sent me for tests, he said he thought my symptoms suggested I might have a brain tumour. As I'd had cancer before, this seemed all too likely, and I spent the week before the appointment reading medical books which all seemed to confirm his suspicions. My children were then in their early teens, and all I could think of was how they would manage if I died. So when, after the MRI scan and various other investigations, we were told that I'd actually got MS, my husband and I went home and opened a bottle of champagne!'*

Even in this situation, however, any sense of relief can only be temporary and disappears as the truth starts to sink in. Some people say that the diagnosis is comparable to the death of someone seriously ill: even though you may have been expecting the news, it is still a shock when it comes. And finding that you have MS may feel like a bereavement in other respects too. What you have lost is your 'healthy self' and it's natural to respond to the loss as a kind of death. The sense of shock may be so powerful that it overwhelms all other feelings, so you remain stunned, disbelieving and unable to take in what is happening to you. At this stage, you may not feel like talking to anyone – neither the doctors nor those closest to you. Julia Segal, a counsellor with many years' experience of working with people with MS, says: 'It takes around two years for the mind to catch up with the body – and this "catching up" process may have to be gone through several times as the condition changes.'

Helena: *'Soon after I was diagnosed, I talked to a woman with MS who told me that the first two years are the hardest. I've just passed my "second anniversary" and that's been one of the most useful pieces of advice anyone has given me.'*

Most of us don't give much thought to good health while we have it – we simply take it for granted. When you are given a diagnosis of MS, anger and resentment are normal reactions. You may feel that life has been unfair – 'Why me?' – and that you need to rage against the injustice of it all. The idea that your life will be restricted by physical limitations, at least some of the time, and that MS may have to be taken into account in any plans you make for the future is daunting and depressing. Most people have to try to deal with all these new emotions while also experiencing symptoms of MS. This makes it even harder to sort out what you're really thinking and feeling. You probably make it more difficult still if you try to do it alone. Talking about your feelings to other people can help to relieve the pressure – some of the possibilities are discussed later in this chapter.

There may be days when you wake up thinking the whole thing has just been a particularly horrible nightmare and that it's not really true. You may even wonder whether the doctors could have got it wrong or be angry with them because they can offer you no cure or even tell you what to expect over the coming months and years.

This process of acknowledging and accepting the reality is a long one for most people, and some would say it never really ends. You need to allow yourself time to get through this emotional turmoil – it is natural and normal to experience confusion and distress before you can really start living again.

LOOKING FOR LOGIC

In an attempt to reduce the chaos which enters their lives with MS, many people try to find patterns or explanations for what is happening to them. Sometimes it helps to make sense of past events and experiences. You may be able to look back on bouts of ill-health or other physical difficulties which were not satisfactorily explained at the time, and realize that they were due to the then undiagnosed MS.

> **Jenny**: *'I'm a naturally energetic person, but for years I've walked more slowly than everyone else, and the last time I tried to ride a bike on a family holiday I just kept losing my balance and fell off several times. At the time I felt really stupid, but now I'm sure it was because of the MS.'*

Sometimes it is possible to begin to recognize factors which have a bearing both on your symptoms and how you react to them. Many people come to know that there are triggers which can bring a worsening of symptoms, and we'll be looking at those in chapter 7. Equally, however, you can look so hard for clues of this kind that you end up following blind alleys. You can't control the way your symptoms come and go, although you may be able to influence your own reactions to them. To take a few examples, eating the 'wrong' foods, going out in the rain or doing 'too much' won't affect the course of the illness. Many people say, though, that factors like this affect how they feel, aggravating their symptoms or making them more noticeable for a while. Getting too warm or overtired is especially likely to cause trouble. Similarly, your mood and your attitude to your MS can't directly affect the course it takes. Feeling cheerful and relaxed has no more bearing on the amount and speed of demyelination you experience than being irritable or un-happy, although of course life in general is more enjoyable when you're in a positive rather than a negative frame of mind.

DENYING REALITY

Once they begin coming out of the initial shock phase, some people react by trying to carry on as though nothing has changed. It's almost as if, by not acknowledging the truth, they can make it go away. This attitude can show itself in a number of ways: refusing to talk about MS, telling no one who doesn't already know and refusing to compromise even when symptoms make carrying on regardless difficult or impractical. (Of course, deciding who and when to tell is a question with wider implications which we'll be considering in detail later.) Some people find it so hard to accept that they have MS that they simply refuse to believe it and convince themselves that the doctors have got it wrong.

Sometimes, family and friends who do know the diagnosis collude with this behaviour, perhaps because they're going along with what they believe to be the wishes of the person with MS, perhaps because they can't face the truth themselves. Alternatively, they may refuse or be unable to take in the reality of the condition. This makes them likely to minimize the symptoms, or suggest that the person with MS can turn them on and off to suit their convenience – 'He can walk well enough when it suits him.' Sometimes they will appear with details of a 'miracle cure' or patent remedy – 'I've heard of these special boots that would mean you could walk properly.' This kind of thing is understandable, but not much help. At its worst, it can develop into a kind of 'blame the victim' attitude: that somehow having MS is your fault, or that you would not have the symptoms if you behaved differently.

A discussion between between people with MS conducted on the Internet included a list of some of the more familiar suggestions offered by supposedly well-meaning people to those with MS. They say that you would get better if only:

- You could get in touch with your inner feelings.
- You could get in touch with your higher powers.
- You stopped fighting yourself and let your body heal itself.
- You really wanted to be well.
- You found Jesus (or Buddha or Allah or . . .)
- You tried the new miracle compound X (or Y or Z or W or . . .)
- You would reduce the stress in your life.
- You were more spiritual.
- You followed the teachings of Eastern mysticism which has all the answers.
- You followed the teachings of Western mysticism which has all the answers.
- You enrolled (with substantial cost) in the clinic of Dr Duck who is persecuted by the orthodox medical

establishment because he is the only one to have real treatments that give good (but unproven) results with therapies involving ———— (some of which sound dangerous, but all of which have very little biological justification).

- You were more active.
- You would eat more.
- You would eat less.
- You would eat healthier food according to the book by Dr X.
- You would meditate.
- You would visualize yourself well.

Mostly, responses like this reflect other people's feelings of helplessness or their desire to find a solution to what seems an insuperable problem. We've all become so used to the idea that good health is our right and that medicine has an answer for every ill that we simply can't accept the fact that it isn't always so.

Facing the fear

However much you learn about MS, you can't find out how it's going to affect you. This fear of the unknown can make it very hard to think straight and make realistic plans about how you will live with the condition. Some people react by simply refusing to think about the future, dealing with their symptoms as best they can when the need arises. Others have said that it was only when they seriously considered what could be in store that they were able to control the fear. Imagining what for them would be the worst that could happen allowed them to think about how they would cope, what help would be available and what preparations they wanted to make. For them, this was less frightening than an unfocused worry which led nowhere.

Of course, there's no right or wrong way to tackle the fear that inevitably accompanies a diagnosis of MS, only the way that's best for you. Acknowledging it and finding a way to counter it is, however, worthwhile if you can do it. Otherwise, you can find yourself mentally and emotionally paralysed by feelings of panic and foreboding so that your life becomes unnecessarily restricted.

> **Frances:** *'I actually think I've become a stronger person since my diagnosis. I rest more and plan what I'm going to do so that I don't get too tired. The secret for me has been learning to live with rather than against my MS.'*

> **Helena:** *'For me, adjusting is an ongoing process, particularly with an unpredictable illness like MS. Thus, MS has taught me how to be flexible. There have been tears, of course, but I have always found other people's reactions more difficult than my own!'*

Testing reactions

As if you didn't have enough to cope with, you may face a whole range of different reactions from the people closest to you. You may not choose to reveal your diagnosis to many outsiders initially, but partners, parents, close friends and perhaps children will be among the first to know. If you are able to share your feelings of grief, anger, fear, depression and anxiety about the future, you may be able to give and gain support from each other. Sadly, this is not always possible, especially at first. In any case, until you have sorted out your own confused responses somewhat, you may not know what you need from those close to you. It's even less likely that you will have compassion and understanding to spare or be able to console anyone else. Like you, other people will need time to take in what has happened and its implications for them as well as for you. Some may want to find out as much as possible about MS, others to bury their heads in the sand. A few may feel like running away – or actually do so, literally or emotionally. Some will want to wrap you in cotton wool, others to pretend that there is nothing seriously wrong. All of these responses are normal and understandable to some degree, but like your own, they are likely to change with time and experience.

Protection

You may have experienced for yourself the consequences of being 'protected' from the truth about your condition. As we saw earlier, doctors are often reluctant to mention MS as a possible diagnosis until they are certain that it is correct. In fact, many people who have suspected the cause of their symptoms were angered and frustrated when doctors refused to confirm their suspicions. Sometimes, the diagnosis is withheld even once it is definite, and relatives are told to keep the secret for fear the person with MS is unable to bear the truth.

Once you do know that you have MS, you are faced with a similar dilemma. You may wonder whether it would be kinder to keep the truth from a child or a parent because it would be too upsetting for them. Of course, only you can make that decision, but it is worth remembering that the people in question will almost certainly be aware that something is wrong. It's possible that the truth might be less frightening or easier to deal with than the explanations they invent for themselves.

Sharing pain

The burden of an MS diagnosis is a heavy one to carry alone. If you are lucky enough to know someone (or perhaps several people) with whom you can talk about your feelings or even sob when you feel like it, it can help to ease the strain. Even though they may not have much to offer in terms of advice, just sharing your feelings without pretence and having someone acknowledge them can be a comfort. If you can't or don't want to talk to someone you know for whatever reason, you might be more comfortable talking to an understanding stranger. The anonymity of the telephone suits some people best, and you'll find the numbers of the helplines run by the MS Society and other organizations on pages 168–70. A few hospitals and many GPs also offer a counselling service, or you could ask your GP to refer you to a psychotherapist. As yet, you may not feel like getting together with other people with MS, but if or when you do, there are numerous support and self-help groups around the country (see page 201–2).

Joining the resistance

It may be just coincidence, but many of those with MS seem to be the type of people who are determined to regain control of their lives and are not willing to become passive 'patients'. Of course, it may just be that it's a question of necessity: when the medical profession can do so little to help, you have to try and help yourself. There is a danger, however, that this can lead you into clutching at straws in the shape of 'quack' cures, some of which do more harm than good. You may also make a big effort to avoid seeing yourself (and being regarded by others) as a 'sick person', but again this can be taken too far. Unless you are willing to recognize the limits your MS places on you, you may be depriving yourself of both the practical and emotional support which could make your life easier. Many people talk in terms of 'beating' MS, refusing to acknowledge that this isn't actually possible. Nothing you do or don't do can, as yet, halt the natural course of the illness, although there's certainly a lot to be gained by making up your mind not to let MS beat you!

> **Sue:** *'I have been fortunate in that my MS tends to affect me in gradually worsening stages, which gives me time to plan ahead for the worse. So far I have been ahead of the game and therefore I remain in control. For example, I got an automatic car before I had no choice and moved to a bungalow before*

stairs became impossible. I am not fighting against MS – it is bigger and stronger than me but I select and win significant battles. I do not exhaust myself doing a "King Canute".'

Taking responsibility

Although the fact that you have MS impinges on the lives of those around you to a greater or lesser extent, you are the one who is most profoundly affected. You have no choice about living with it and only you really know how it feels. Where you do have some choice is in what you do about it – what attitude you adopt towards yourself and your future way of life. Obviously the reactions of other people have a bearing on this and are very important, but it is your own response which is crucial. This doesn't imply that you have to keep a stiff upper lip, minimizing your problems and smiling bravely come what may. Nor does it suggest that your attitude to your MS will make your symptoms milder or easier to bear or that you won't often feel angry, frustrated and sad. What can help is finding your way – probably gradually or even repeatedly – to a balance between what you want and what is possible. If you can see yourself literally as 'a person with MS', you may begin to accept the MS as an inevitable part of your life but one which doesn't always or even often take centre stage.

This may sound like a counsel of perfection – and it's certainly not easy to achieve and maintain such a balance. During a relapse or when existing symptoms become more severe, then the fact that you have MS is bound to dominate your thoughts and feelings. You will have to make adjustments all over again, but many people do manage to do this repeatedly and so achieve some degree of mastery over their MS.

> **Sue**: *'I live with my MS but on my terms. I am the world's expert on how MS affects me. I am not "an MS sufferer", I am a person who happens to have MS. I have MS, MS doesn't have me!'*

How much help?

Even the most sensitive and well-intentioned person can't know what you want from them (if anything) at any given moment. Sometimes, it might be low key, practical help to get round a physical difficulty, sometimes a listening, patient ear, sometimes to behave as though there were nothing wrong. What often happens instead is they will try to give what they think you need or what makes them feel better about your MS. This can range from trying to wrap you in cotton wool and treat you like an invalid, to a brisk, pull-yourself-together breeziness.

There is no way to solve this problem completely, and in any case, your needs change in response to how you feel, both physically and mentally. All you can do is to try to decide what exactly you do want and ask for it directly wherever possible. This means being honest with yourself – do you want special consideration and allowances made for you? Do you want to discuss your symptoms and/or your emotional state? Do you want people to forget or ignore the fact that you have MS most of the time? Of course there is no categorical answer to such questions, but your responses will depend on how you see the role of MS in your life as a whole. You may want help and support when you have new symptoms or existing ones worsen, or when you're feeling very down, but otherwise prefer not to be treated as someone who's ill. On the other hand, you may need others to acknowledge your condition, and not expect you to behave as you did before you developed MS. If you can clarify such things in your own mind, it will help you to make any necessary adjustments in your relationships with other people, even though there will always be some whose attitudes and behaviour are immovable.

ACCEPTING HELP

If you're someone who's always been independent and self-reliant, accepting help, even when you need it, is one of the hardest things. For many people, being able to acknowledge that they can sometimes do with a helping hand is a measure of how far they have accepted the reality of MS. It means accepting that the condition imposes certains limitations on your activity, but not that you have become a different person as a consequence. The fact that you find it a struggle to carry a tray of tea or reach a plug at ground level says nothing about you as a person. You'd do better to save your energy for things that really matter and let other people deal with such trivial inconveniences. Of course, this assumes that they are aware of your physical difficulties, whether or not they know the reason for them. However, it isn't necessary to give a full medical history before asking for a minor favour. 'I've done my back in – would you mind plugging in the computer please' will usually do perfectly well for a colleague or acquaintance whom you prefer to keep in the dark.

When your disability is obvious, you may sometimes be plagued by people trying to force help on you or doing exactly the wrong thing. A sensitive person will ask you whether there is anything they can do to assist, but it's not always easy to fend off the one who grabs hold of your arm or your bag when you only need them to open a door. Some people just learn to put up with this kind of thing on the grounds that it's well-meant. The alternative does require some assertiveness in making it clear what you do and don't need, but you may feel it's worth the effort!

Further down the road

Whatever thoughts and feelings you have now about your MS, your perspective will change with time. As we have seen, many people cope initially by doing all they can to ignore the fact that they have MS, while others embark on frantic searches for a cure or believe they will conquer the illness if only they fight it with enough determination. These tactics don't work indefinitely, so eventually there has to be some acknowledgement that MS is here to stay. That doesn't necessarily imply 'acceptance' – a word which is pretty meaningless in the context of MS. Feelings of anger and resentment remain prominent for some people, while others do enjoy happy and fulfilling lives, despite MS. A few can even say that they can identify a good side to having MS and that it has brought gains they might otherwise have missed.

Hazel: *'Before I knew I had MS, I remember occasional bouts of depression and weeping at the incomprehensible sensations I* *experienced. When I finally discovered what it was, the truth came as a great relief. I immediately went to the library and read up on MS so I knew what to expect. It became a ludicrous game, battling with each ridiculous symptom as it came – such as burning, numbness, problems of balance, swallowing and most physical processes. Fortunately for me, not much pain – I just collapse in a heap.*

'I trained as a primary school teacher and managed for a year, in spite of minor MS symptoms. After having had three children myself, I had to give up full-time teaching as I could only last half a day before exhaustion took over. I retired but opened a small nursery school in my home which ran for 25 years. Mornings only – then collapse into bed pm! I had to divide my time between living and resting. When my physical activity was curtailed by MS in the 1970s, I sat on the floor and travelled far in books, ending up with a BA Hons degree from the Open University. It was great fun and I would recommend any of the myriad OU courses to people with MS because they make all sorts of timing allowances for you.

'When I needed it, I got marvellous help from parents, husband and family and the social services. MS is impossible when you don't have this. A reasonable amount of money also helps – my husband has a steady job and pay packet. It is easier for the comparatively rich to be disabled. If you are poor and badly hit, MS is the pits.'

Valerie: *'I had to give up working when I was 39 – it was awful. Then I thought that so much of what you are is your job. I dreaded meeting people socially who were bound to ask "What do you do?" Not only that, but I had a mortgage on my own – something I was proud of and I liked living alone. I thought I would be hopeless and helpless and I was really afraid I might end up in the gutter. I don't have a large family, and anyway they weren't in a position to help very much. For ages I went around thinking "I'll do that when I'm* *better," and I went through a severe depression when I finally realized I wasn't going to get better. I held little discussions with myself, and decided I had to do something – I wasn't 38 any more. I made lists of things to achieve – silly little things sometimes – and felt triumphant when I crossed them off. I know now what I can do on good days and bad days – and that sometimes I'll pay the price of a week's exhaustion if I do too much. I do it anyway, and don't tell anyone, otherwise they'd want to stop me. I know what to do. I'm not accepting – I hate that word – but I am philosophical. I've had to draw on resources I didn't know I had and I actually think I'm a better person because of the MS. I'm glad I've had the experience of delving into myself. I'm more realistic now, less romantic and I say what I really think.'*

Ann: *'After the initial shock of discovering I had MS came a slow, sometimes interrupted but sometimes satisfying process of acceptance and accommodation. I am not seriously disabled and I feel I have been given a kind of second chance. I have an excuse to let go of much unimportant clutter and personal ambition.'*

Of course, it would be unrealistic and unfair to imply that everyone who has MS can or should be able to focus on the positive in this way. For some, MS still seems an unmitigated disaster – a cloud which has no silver lining.

Janet: *'I hate having MS – it's taken away my energy and messed up my life. The only thing which would make my life better is not having it. I wish I could be a strong and positive disabled person, the sort you read about and hear on the radio, but I can't.'*

99

Counselling

Ideally, counselling should be automatically offered to everyone with MS. If this were to happen at the time of diagnosis, some people would accept it immediately, some would reject the idea completely. Others would welcome the opportunity to talk to a counsellor at different points, perhaps soon after initial diagnosis or when they feel they are facing a crisis of some kind. Julia Segal, one of the few counsellors with extensive experience of working with people with MS, says people often choose to come when other events in their lives are making the MS unbearable. The pressure can come from any sphere, but will make itself felt in a person's most vulnerable areas – whether these are relationships with a partner, family, friends or colleagues or the way the person regards him- or herself.

For example, one of the first and most important pressure points for many people is when the symptoms of MS begin to threaten their livelihood. The prospect that you will lose the ability to do your job threatens not just your material well-being, but also undermines your self-image. For many of us, what we do is closely tied into how we see ourselves and how we think others see us. After all, when we're introduced to strangers, one of the first pieces of information we exchange is often what we do (or used to do or plan to do) for a living.

In this situation, a counsellor might encourage you to explore anger, distress, fears for the future and how you might reconcile your former self-image with your image of yourself as a person with MS. Sometimes, there are lots of different strands that must be unravelled before you can begin finding a way to deal with them. Julia Segal points out that you can't think about 'coming to terms with MS' until and unless you define what MS is to you. Your MS is different from anyone else's, not just because symptoms vary, but in every respect, so your way of living with it will be unique too. A counsellor will try to help you work out what your way might be and how you can negotiate the obstacles in your path – both now and in the future.

Sometimes it is hard to separate the physical from psychological elements in the difficulties thrown your way by MS. This can be worth attempting because you may be able to modify the way you feel and think even though you cannot get rid of the symptom itself. For example, many people resist using a wheelchair even though they can barely get about. It is as if the symbolism attached to becoming a wheelchair user is so negative that it outweighs the mobility advantages. There are genuine reasons why this should be so, yet the problem is partly one of perception. While it is true that the wheelchair does have unfortunate associations in the minds of many people, using one does not change you as a person. What it may well do, however, is make you feel differently about yourself – many people talk of wheelchairs in terms of 'giving in'. A counsellor may help you to separate your feelings about the loss of your mobility from your hostility to the idea of a wheelchair, caused by its negative associations. In this way, you can grieve for your real loss without rejecting a way of counteracting that loss. For some people, talking with a counsellor is the only time when they feel free to express their grief, anger and anxiety without covering up. They feel – often, although not always correctly – that those close to them couldn't cope with these feelings. The opportunity to bring them into the open in a controlled situation with a 'neutral' person can come as a real relief. It also offers the chance to identify, and face up to, your worst fears so you can get them into perspective and find ways of coping with them. In her booklet 'Emotional reactions to MS', Julia Segal quotes some comments from people whom she has counselled:

'When I came to you six months ago, MS was the biggest thing in my life. Now it's sort of taken its place with other things, it's not the main thing any more. You made me look at it differently. Since we talked about it I've been able to tell people about it, and their reactions have been quite different from what I expected. They have made me change my life. I'm doing things I want to do now.'

'I was very angry after talking to you last week. You made me face it all – well, I made myself really. But I hadn't wanted to . . . except that that was why I came. By the middle of the week, I felt much better than I had before, and I said to my sister "I can see why the Americans go for this sort of thing."'

Professional help can open up new avenues and show you different ways of pursuing the 'fight' against MS.

Helena: *'I was given no counselling when I was first diagnosed, but eventually a trainee GP referred me to a cognitive behavioural therapist after I began to lose my mobility. The psychologist was very helpful. She helped me to let go of my 'old' life and to embrace the positive in my life with MS . . . It's hard to explain to others that fighting MS can sometimes mean giving in. Where fatigue is concerned, for example, you just can't keep fighting in a physical sense. But if you're not seen to be fighting physically, then it's assumed you've given up. I prefer to seek to accommodate my MS rather than to battle against it. MS is more of a friend and teacher to me than my enemy.'*

6

YOU AND YOUR RELATIONSHIPS

Dealing with Change

Any sudden and major alteration in our lives – especially when it's not good news – will shed new and surprising light on our relationships with other people. This happens to people who are bereaved, whose financial circumstances alter dramatically, who go through a traumatic experience such as a plane crash, as well as to those who develop a serious illness. Sometimes it's those you thought you could rely on who let you down, while others surprise you by turning into a tower of strength. Many people have commented that 'you really find out who your friends are when you have MS'.

Sadly, many people with MS say they have lost friends or experienced broken relationships as a direct result of having the condition. There are all kinds of reasons for this, but even when you can understand them, it's still hard to take. Although your MS may have in some way triggered these changes, it's worth bearing in mind that you would probably have lost some of these people anyway in the normal course of events. For example, you might find that you have less in common with a friend you made at work after one of you leaves. Once the cement of shared experience is gone, there's little to hold you together and your friendship fades naturally away. But if you left for health reasons, it's easy to assume that any cooling off has occurred because your MS has come between you. It can also be harder to tolerate other people's imperfections because you become more sensitive. A friend whose tactless remarks were always something of a joke can seem far from funny when their comments are targeted at your more vulnerable spots.

While those who knew you 'before' can certainly alter, those you meet for the first time as a person with MS can react to you in ways you never encountered before. People do stare, make comments or just ignore you completely. You are likely to be given all manner of unwanted advice or subjected to uninvited and misguided attempts to 'help'. Ironically, this can be a particular nuisance if your disability doesn't happen to be immediately obvious to other people.

> **Helena:** *'I have an orange badge in my car, and obviously I park in the special parking bays quite often. I'm always getting people knocking on the window informing me that I'm in a parking space reserved for people with disabilities. Usually, I just smile and thank them for telling me. Sometimes, they'll keep on, but of course, their faces change when I get out with my stick or unload my wheelchair.'*

There are some who will tell you that this kind of thing isn't your problem: if strangers or casual acquaintances have difficulties dealing with the fact that you have MS, that's for them to worry about. That may be true, strictly speaking, but it can make going out more of an ordeal than it need be. Few of us are able to ignore other people's reactions completely, and can't help getting upset or embarrassed by them at times.

When we make a fool of ourselves in public – say by spilling a glass of wine or tripping over – we tend to feel it's because we've been careless or clumsy. It was our own fault and might have been avoided. When something like this happens because you have MS, the situation is different because you are not responsible in the same sense. If you fall because your sense of balance is disturbed or your legs won't obey you, it is the MS which is responsible, not you as a person. Other people won't necessarily know this, but you do and the distinction is important. You have enough to do getting over the problems which MS creates for you without worrying about what strangers think. If you are brave enough to continue going out into the world despite your physical difficulties, why get upset about something so trivial as a funny look or ignorant comment from someone you don't know?

Those people who manage not to lose their sense of humour find it can serve them well in what would otherwise be intolerable situations. You may not often be able to see anything funny in the various indignities MS forces upon you, but for those who can, humour is an important weapon in their battle for psychological equilibrium.

Jenny: *'I had parked my car on a main road outside the office with the passenger door next to the kerb. I was finding walking a real struggle that day, so I decided to get into the car on that side. My friend then helped me to try and shift across into the driving seat, and as she forced my unbending legs* *across the gear lever, we suddenly caught sight of the expressions of the people in the bus queue on the other side of the street. They looked so gobsmacked at seeing this wrestling match taking place between two middle-aged women that we just collapsed in giggles and neither of us could do anything useful until we recovered.'*

Hazel: *'I get a lot of help from my relatives, which enables me to treat most of it as the joke it is. How else?'*

Naturally, life would be pleasanter if you encountered nothing but understanding and a genuinely helpful attitude from the rest of the world, but this will never be the case. Nevertheless, people will often be pleased to help once they know what's needed. Restaurants will keep you a table near the entrance, shop assistants will let you use the staff loo if it's more accessible and drivers will wait patiently while you slowly cross the road if you make your requirements clear. Not every time, maybe, but mostly. If you're not embarrassed or apologetic, other people are less likely to be so as well. It's unfair that you should have to allow for other people's hang-ups as well as coping with your own symptoms, but if you can manage to appear confident and assertive, it often makes a big difference. You might call it the 'Does she take sugar?' syndrome: a person with an obvious physical disability may be defined by it unless the power of their personality can force others to see the individual instead of just the disability. This approach comes naturally to a few people, and some others start to adopt it out of sheer impatience and frustration. You can end up coming straight out with what you want to say in many situations simply because the polite, roundabout approach gets you absolutely nowhere! Whatever the difficulties, dealing with the wider world is likely to be child's play compared to sorting out your relationships with people close to you. Both your feelings and theirs will be complex and changeable, and in some cases you are likely to face real problems for which there are no easy answers.

You and your partner

A marriage or partnership does not run on tramlines – it is subject to change and adaptation over time and as circumstances alter. This is true for everyone, but MS can (and usually does) impose extra pressures on the relationship. Sadly, separation and divorce are not uncommon when one of the partners has MS, although some of these relationships would have broken up anyway. If you and your partner got together at a time when you already knew that you had MS, you may feel that you are prepared for the changes which your condition may force on you in the future. Nevertheless, such changes and the way you each respond to them may throw up problems you hadn't allowed for. On the other hand, if the diagnosis came later, you both have to come to terms with the shock and the fact that the future is likely to be different from the one you expected to share.

Martin: *I'm now going through a divorce, and I'm certain that my MS has been a major contributory factor in our marital difficulties. I hate having it. I hope that I am slowly coming to terms with it, but I do feel bitter that, aged only 20, I began to experience the symptoms of MS. I feel now that I* *should have sought some counselling years ago, before my bitterness and loss of self-respect wrecked my marriage.'*

To have the best chance of helping one another and cementing your relationship, you need to be able to talk and understand one another's feelings. This assumes that you're both the kind of people who are willing and able to do this, but not everyone is like that. Either or both of you may be the strong silent type, finding it difficult or impossible to put your emotions into words. And if there were already problems in your relationship, the stresses caused by MS can crack the fault lines wide open. Communication can easily break down, leaving you both feeling isolated and alone. Alternatively, it may have the effect of making you concentrate on problems which you'd previously chosen to ignore.

Chloe: *'I have no real idea about how my diagnosis affected my partner although he did leave me, but for reasons other than MS, I think. He knew about the possibility right from the start but did not want to talk about what it might mean for us, other than to say "It won't happen to you." When I asked him whether he was leaving because I had MS, he said: "What? Oh no, I haven't really thought about it." It hardly affected him on a practical level, except when he had to cook and wash up for a couple of months when I lost the use of my hand, but I have no idea how it affected him emotionally.*

'I'm feeling very pessimistic about relationships now, which I suppose isn't surprising as I'm in the middle of a break-up. I feel I'm a walking time bomb and that no man in his right mind would consider getting involved with me. If I should start dating, when should I tell them I have MS? I don't even feel up to telling all of my friends yet!'

It's not unusual for the person with MS to try – consciously or unconsciously – to push their partner away. Often this comes from a feeling that no one should be expected to share the burden of MS and that the only fair course of action is to give a partner their freedom. 'Who wants to be tied for life to someone like me?' The feeling is that, regardless of what he or she may say to the contrary, they're just being kind.

Sometimes, it has to be said, this really is the case. For whatever reason, some people simply cannot cope with the prospect of staying with a partner who has a condition such as MS. They may actually decide to leave or perhaps to withdraw from any real closeness and intimacy. Occasionally it happens the other way around. When a relationship has been unsatisfactory for some time, the person with MS may be the one who decides that fixing it or continuing to put up with it is a waste of valuable energy.

Helena: *'My original partner left in horror. My new partner is supportive but wants me to "defeat" MS. However, I don't really mind having it – it's part of me.'*

Sue: *'I had an on/off relationship, but with MS I decided to put myself first and permanently "offed" him. I've had no second thoughts. At times I think it would be interesting to swap my Disability Living Allowance Personal Care Component for a strong but gentle bloke – provided of course I could swap him back for the money if I changed my mind!'*

Robin: *'I don't yet have a full-time partner, and many girlfriends have left me because of my MS. I've had two short-lived engagements, both of which I ended because of my uncertainty about the future. I'm fed up with being single* *and would love to be married. I returned to my second fiancée after five months because I missed her and her children. Maybe we might get re-engaged, but I don't think so because my professional, well-salaried career isn't there any more.'*

It's probably only a minority of couples who give up on their relationship almost immediately. While it's impossible to generalize about what happens to those who don't, many will find themselves facing the same issues. Top of many couples' lists is anger. It isn't the emotion itself, but how it is directed and expressed which is potentially destructive. Indeed, it would be strange if angry feelings weren't on show or just barely suppressed a lot of the time. MS gives both partners plenty of good reasons to rage – against the condition, its effect on their lives and against themselves and each other. It's important to recognize and be open about the real source of anger and its target. For example, it's easy to turn on your partner for failing to offer the right kind of help at the right moment when what's really making you furious is the fact that you need help at all. Most of us have a tendency to hit out at the nearest target when we can't get at the real culprit. If both partners know that this is the reason for frequent angry outbursts, it can make them easier to live with and less likely to be taken personally.

Some couples do actually manage to see the MS as a kind of 'third party' in their relationship. It is separate from both of them, but exerts all kinds of pressures which neither person can be 'blamed' for, but which they each have to deal with. By constructing this fiction, they can go on as if nothing has changed between them, even though MS has altered their circumstances. Yet people who perceive their MS as a part of who they are would find such an approach unacceptable, in that it denies a part of their reality. For them, a successful relationship must take account of the fact of MS and work outwards from it.

The point is that there are as many ways of tackling MS within a relationship as there are couples, and no one can offer a blueprint for doing it successfully. It's not unusual for the person who has MS to feel that they shouldn't burden their partner with all the details of their worries and symptoms. If you feel you can cope, more or less, it may seem easier to get on with it rather than having to deal with someone else's concern as well.

Sarah: *'My husband is aware of my MS, but as I go attack-free for many years at a time, I think he is "comfortable" with it. However, he does panic and become extremely worried and protective when I tell him about any new numbness. The numbnesses seem to come and go, so I tend to keep them to myself so he doesn't get worried too.'*

Where there are real difficulties, all relationship counsellors stress the point that nothing can be resolved unless both partners share their feelings clearly and honestly. And sharing means what it says – listening properly when your partner has his or her say as well as expressing your own concerns and being listened to in return. No one is suggesting that this is easy, but unless you can communicate, your relationship is almost bound to suffer. When two people haven't been in the habit of keeping in close touch with one another's feelings, MS may provide a good reason to begin. You may well discover all sorts of things about one another which you never knew before. Whether your relationship improves as a result only experience will reveal.

When opening up and expressing difficult emotions for the first time, many couples find it helps to be in a structured setting such as a counselling session. A neutral person can help keep the discussion on track and make it easier for each partner to hear what the other is saying without losing emotional control. Counsellors, such as those from Relate, are trained to help couples find their own way through their problems rather than proffering any ready-made solutions. Even if you or your partner are wary of counselling, it could be worth giving the idea serious thought if your relationship is struggling. It is unlikely to do any harm, and you may find it more use than you'd expected.

Whether you do it alone or with help, opening clear lines of communication with your partner will give you a better chance of dealing with other difficulties in your relationship. One which is likely to keep recurring in different forms is any shift in emotional and 'lifestyle' balance forced on you by one partner's MS. For example, one may have always held the domestic fort while the other concentrated on a career, or maybe one of you relied on the other to take the social lead – organizing parties, arranging outings and holidays, seeing family and friends. Whatever was the set-up before, MS can mean you have to change arrangements which suited you both, give up old responsibilities or take on new ones. This can be extremely upsetting, especially if you never really thought much about how things worked before, or why.

Jenny: *'My husband was always ambitious, and as his career took off, I was quite happy to put mine on hold while the children were young. He worked long hours and travelled a lot, and I ran the house and organized our social life, and enjoyed having people round all the time. I really hated it when my MS wouldn't let me do everything I'd always done –*

I didn't want my husband to help with the cooking and insisted on doing the supermarket shopping even when it got really difficult. From his point of view, he started worrying about me when he had to go away for work, and felt guilty and resentful. Before he could just go knowing I could cope quite happily. Now I can't, and that makes me angry. I've never been the dependent type and I can't get used to it.'

The adjustments necessitated by MS may generate a fair amount of friction. You may find it difficult to recognize when you can no longer manage a particular task as you used to. Your partner, on the other hand, can become frustrated or angry when you insist on struggling rather than accept help. Such situations can become a battle between one person's determination not to 'give in' and the other's impatience with what they perceive as stubbornness or sheer bloody-mindedness. Unless you are able to recognize when this is happening and try to stop it, hostilities may continue to break out at regular intervals. If you are able to identify the real cause of the conflict and begin fighting on the same side, you stand a better chance of keeping your relationship close and strong.

This assumes that it really is MS which is responsible for your difficulties. You might, of course, come to see the condition more as a catalyst – provoking a reaction which would have come eventually, albeit more slowly. In other words, you may realize that if it hadn't been for the MS, you'd have ended up rowing over sex, money or something else.

Whether or not that is the case, MS can be the make-or-break factor in a relationship that might otherwise have gone either way. The problem of adapting is compounded by the need to enter into fresh negotiations as symptoms fluctuate and alter the picture. It is often hard for both partners to distinguish between behaviour which is the direct result of demyelination and that which is a reflection of an individual's psyche and thus affected by many other things besides MS. In reality, suffering rarely turns people into saints, and you may well be more short-tempered and selfish, less considerate and thoughtful than you once were because you have MS. It's also possible that some of your responses may be influenced by neurological changes which have subtle effects on your personality. Trying to disentangle physical from purely psychological causes is probably a waste of time. However, it's important for both partners to be aware that such changes may occur as a result of MS, and are under no more voluntary control than a stiff leg. Depression, over-the-top optimism, emotional volatility, forgetfulness and sudden mood swings are some of the more common features of MS which can be caused by changes in the CNS. Like other symptoms, they can come and go but because they seem to affect the essence of a person, their personality, a partner may find them harder to cope with than clear-cut physical symptoms.

Paul: *I have read about personality changes associated with MS, and always assumed these resulted from certain kinds of localized brain damage and, as far as anyone can comment objectively about their own personality, I would insist that I have not been so affected. However, I am sure that my wife would say that I have become more stubborn, selfish, inconsiderate, lazy and self-pitying of late. I won't deny this, but I also suspect it is a common reaction of people who suddenly find their aspirations in jeopardy in some way. I suppose it can be summarised as a sudden feeling of dissatisfaction with all sorts of aspects of one's life, coupled with a panic that time may be running out to do anything* *about it. And, to put it crudely, it has elements of "my body has decided to give me a hard time, so I don't see why I should take it from anything or anyone else."*

'My wife and I have always had different priorities regarding what makes for a satisfying life. She wants to spend our savings on travel, which I'm happy to go along with. However, there are other things I want to do while I still can, many of which might be seen as a nostalgia for lost youth (is this the male menopause?). My wife works hard at her job, and is so badly affected by disputes with our adolescent son that she often just wants quiet evenings and early nights. My wishes, on the other hand, are to continue to make use of my energy while I still have it, in the selfish pursuit of happiness. Before my diagnosis I would have thought: "Perhaps things will change for the better in a few years' time when our son has left home." Now, my thoughts are more on the lines of: "What good will it be if things do change for the better, but I'm stuck in a wheelchair?" At the moment, I am still able to justify this egocentricity to myself, but I don't know if it is the first step towards a permanent change of personality. I don't want to end up a sort of Victor Meldrew, self-obsessed, intolerant and permanently complaining. Neither do I wish, cynically, to hang on to an unsatisfying relationship as an insurance against a lonely old age.'

When a relationship is going wrong for whatever reason, it's likely that a couple's sex life will suffer too. Sexual difficulties are extremely common, and by assuming MS is behind them, you may be missing the real problem. That isn't to say, of course, that MS may not be a contributing factor. For some couples it may really be the main obstacle to a happy sex life. Physical restrictions which make movement awkward or painful, or the effect of MS on the normal functioning of the sexual organs are the obvious culprits, but many couples are able to find ways around such difficulties. Aids such as jelly for vaginal lubrication, vibrators and other 'sex toys' can play a part. A willingness to experiment sexually – sometimes necessarily combined with a sense of humour – enables many couples to continue enjoying a fulfilling sex life, even though 'normal' sexual intercourse is difficult or impossible because of one partner's MS. Someone who's concerned about incontinence may get into the habit of always visiting the loo before starting to make love or need to get specialist advice about a catheter, for example. The point here is that, even if the physical symptoms of MS do impinge on your sex life, it doesn't automatically mean that it must change for the worse.

Subtler, less obvious factors are sometimes harder to recognize and resolve. Either or both of you may find that MS has altered the way you relate to each other or built up barriers between you – and this is bound to have some effect on your sexual relationship. The symptoms of MS may well have given your self-image quite a battering, and some people find it hard to go on seeing themselves as sexually desirable. They may react by pushing their partner away in the belief they can't really want to make love or by going to the opposite extreme and demanding constant sexual reassurance. Even if the person with MS has no such emotional hang-ups, their partner may well have others. At it simplest, there may be the fear of causing pain or discomfort or somehow aggravating the symptoms of MS. This shouldn't be too difficult to sort out, especially once you both accept that sexual activity can't exacerbate MS – the worst that can happen is a bout of fatigue which may make any symptoms more obvious for a day or so. It can be more difficult if the demands of the illness edge you into playing the roles of nurse and patient rather than lovers. Some couples are able to incorporate whatever physical caring is necessary into their relationship without losing their sexual intimacy. This isn't possible for everyone, and many people prefer that their partner doesn't adopt the dual role of carer as well.

The fact that sexual problems are so common means that there is professional help available, although services may be scarcer in some areas than others. Psychosexual counsellors practise both privately and within the NHS, although many may have had no experience of clients with MS. Advice and counselling are also available from SPOD – The Association to Aid the Sexual and Personal Relationships of People with a Disability, 286 Camden Road, London N7 0BJ; tel: 0171 607 8851. There is a counselling service available on this number on Tuesdays (10.30 am to 13.30 pm, Wednesdays 13.30 pm to 16.30 pm and Thursdays 10.30 am to 13.30 pm). They also have a range of advice leaflets including 'Multiple Sclerosis and Sex' and 'Sex and Incontinence', price 50p each.

All this may have made you feel that it is virtually impossible for a relationship to survive MS, but of course this is far from being the case. Current statistics show that one in three marriages (and a higher proportion of second and subsequent ones) end in divorce, and many which survive go through temporary bad patches. In the majority of cases, MS is clearly not a factor. People with MS are no different even though the break-up rate is probably higher, but that still means that very many, probably the majority, of marriages and partnerships do last.

> **Graeme**: *'In some ways we are closer now and have a stronger relationship. On the other hand, I have days when I get moody and short-tempered and this puts a strain on us. It led to a crisis point, but we are over it now.'*

Hazel Chesterman-Phillips was diagnosed as having MS in 1952, when she was 17, although she was told it was 'neuralgia' and 'spasm' and only discovered the truth ten years later.

'It was all rather hushed up and feared in those days. My father, who was a Harley Street specialist, gave my husband-to-be a rather grim prognosis, but he married me anyway! His attitude to MS was liberal, like my parents', and he has been (and still is) steadfast and brill, as they say nowadays. We've had three children, now all grown up, and I followed my husband as his job took him all round the world. I am lucky that I have been able to keep going, albeit at a slow pace. The worst of it has fallen on my husband, who regularly has to pick up the pieces and take over when I fade out from time to time. He has just this minute picked me up from the kitchen floor where I fell, trying to reach something from a high cupboard. Nigel explodes in exasperation sometimes, but he is always my lifeline.'

Children

The effect a parent's MS has on a child will depend on the severity of the illness, on relationships within the family and on other factors unique to each individual. In any case, it will change with time as the child grows older. Having said that, it is possible to pinpoint some elements which seem to be common to many families and which influence relationships within them. Knowing your own child (or children) better than anyone else, you will be the best judge of how much they need to be told about MS at each stage. While no one would want to over-burden children with too much information or detail which disturbed them, there is a risk of leaning too far the other way. If a parent suddenly develops new and serious symptoms or has to go into hospital, a child may well need a fairly full explanation of what's happening. You may need to talk quite a lot about the changes which MS brings, both for the parent him- or herself and for everyone else. It may seem obvious to adults, but children often need to be reassured that they are not responsible for the MS or for making it worse. A child who knows that their parent only developed (or found out about) MS after their birth may assume they must have 'caused' the illness. Similarly, if a relapse happens to follow an argument or even a session of rough play, a child may blame him- or herself unless someone thinks to explain that there is no connection between the two things.

Children are often very quick to sense emotional atmospheres and are aware of all kinds of currents which parents imagine pass over their heads. While they may not fully understand the basis of it, they will respond to tension or an air of secrecy and mistrust between you and your partner. It's also not unknown for them to exploit any apparent divisions between you for their own ends. Of course, this happens in all families, but there is likely to be extra scope where there are unresolved issues between parents because one has MS. For example, it may be that the threat of causing a relapse is used as a means of control – by either or both parents. It may be done overtly where the child is told specifically that upsetting the parent with MS will make their symptoms worse. It can also be simply assumed from the behaviour of the adults even though no one ever spells it out. Alternatively, the child may pick up quite a different message – that the parent with MS could actually control their symptoms and do more if they wanted to.

It's not that anyone is consciously trying to colour the child's view of the true situation. Manipulation is frequently more or less a by-product of the reactions experienced and expressed by his or her parents. When you're struggling with emotional issues thrown up by MS, it can be hard to remember that your children may feel directly involved in the difficulties being faced by you. They may believe that they are responsible for conflicts or for resolving them, however unrealistic this actually is. When tension is high, or during an MS relapse, children sometimes worry about whether their parents will be able to go on looking after them, or what will happen if they can't. You should also be aware that your child may have other questions which might not get asked for fear of the answers. In particular, whether the parent with MS is going to die, and whether the child him- or herself will get MS.

How or whether these concerns show in a child's behaviour will vary: common signs of stress include disruptiveness at school, anxiety, bullying other children or, at the other extreme, behaviour so 'perfect' that it seems (and is) unnatural. Having other family members or friends around can help if they are willing to spend time with the children and do their share of listening and explaining. Sometimes a child finds it easier to talk to someone other than the parents about what's really on his or her mind. For children up the age of around 12, there's a useful booklet from the MS Society 'Has your Mum or Dad got MS?' which covers the common concerns very well. The authors suggest that the child reads it with a parent or other adult or that both read it then talk about any questions or worries the child may have.

It's probably a bit too basic for teenagers, and currently there isn't anything designed specifically for that age group. While their concerns will overlap with those of younger siblings, they may have their own difficulties tied up with normal adolescent angst. Virtually all teenagers are deeply embarrassed by their parents and if you happen to limp or use a wheelchair, it is likely to be that rather than your hair or clothes which makes it impossible for your child to be seen in public with you. The fact that teenagers can be so hurtful and offensive at times means it's difficult, and sometimes impossible, to sympathize with the feelings behind their bad behaviour. Sulks, rudeness and aggression are common enough, but they also make a good cover for pain and insecurity which may in part arise from worry about you and your MS. Convincing you – and hopefully themselves too – that they don't care about you and your problems may leave them free to concentrate on their own. They may be embarrassed or angry that they can't rely on you for certain kinds of help – such as chauffeuring – in the way their friends can rely on their families. They may not like their friends to see you if your disabilities are obvious and discourage you from attending parents' evenings or other school events. It is often hard to know whether or when to intervene and sometimes it is better to let them work things through on their own. Some parents find it helps to compare notes with school staff who know the child well and see him or her in a different context. Many schools now offer student counselling or can arrange it if required.

The urge to separate from their parents is a natural one in adolescents, but it sometimes starts earlier in children who are worried by a parent's disability. Trying to loosen emotional ties and create some distance in their family relationships may be a child's form of self-defence against a range of difficult feelings. It may help if you can bring these out in the open – encouraging your child to talk about how he or she feels, answering questions honestly and repeatedly if necessary and giving as much reassurance as you can that he or she is safe and loved.

> **Paul**: *'When we told our teenage son, he was distressed and supportive for about 30 minutes! He keeps needing to be reminded that I get tired easily and can't always do what he wants.'*

Some children react to uncertainty by trying to turn themselves into little adults – always willing to help and behave sensibly and showing few if any signs of distress. While such willing support may be welcome, it can go too far for the child's emotional well-being. It isn't so healthy, for example, if the adults come to rely on the children in important ways – as part-time carers or as emotional support for either or both parents. If you feel this situation has developed or might do so in your own family, you may be better able to tackle it by calling in some kind of outside assistance. Your GP, social services department, minister of religion or a counsellor are all possible sources of help who can offer professional advice and possibly practical support to relieve the pressure.

It's almost inevitable that your illness will have some bearing on the way things are organized and run at home. When symptoms of MS limit your ability to do housework or other domestic chores, there's no reason why children shouldn't take a share, even at a relatively young age. Having to give a hand earlier in life than some of their friends won't do them any harm, provided what's expected of them is reasonable. You will have your own opinions about how much you think it fair to ask of a child in this respect, and children's protests may bear little relation to how much they are actually asked to do. If you do sometimes suffer pangs of guilt because your condition means they have to help, it's worth remembering that many other children will be expected to do more with less justification.

MS may well take on greater or lesser significance at different periods in family life. You may find it looming larger during times when you are experiencing new or more serious symptoms which require everyone to make fresh adjustments. At other times, it will feel more like a background factor which everyone is used to and so takes more or less for granted. Although it can clearly create real difficulties for some children in some situations, it can also help them to develop greater maturity and understanding of other people's problems.

> **Hazel:** *'My three children are now grown up and have all done well. I think they have sometimes found my MS hard to accept with equanimity but now they pop in to see me whenever their busy lives allow.'*

Parents

For some people with MS, their parents' distress and concern for them feels like one more burden to carry. Some react by trying to hide or minimize their symptoms or maintain a resolutely cheerful demeanour regardless of the true situation. This may seem especially necessary if parents feel that they are to blame in some way for the fact that their child has this condition. They may be very anxious to offer help and support but have little idea of what form this should take. Unless this is sorted out relatively early on, you can end up feeling like a child again and in danger of losing your independence.

As always, the way you work things out will be determined in part by the kind of relationship you had before MS was diagnosed. If you've had to struggle for the right to be yourself and live your own life, you may be reluctant to accept any kind of parental support that could undermine your hard-won freedom. When pleasing your parents has always been important to you, developing MS can feel like 'letting them down' – however ludicrous that is in reality. It's worse still if a parent seems to see it as Cari Loder's did. She has talked of the way her father reacted to learning that she had MS: 'Every time we spoke on the phone, my father constantly told me that I'd broken his heart by getting MS – as though I'd done it to spite him!'

You may also want to protect your parents from suffering on your behalf, especially if they are elderly or in poor health themselves.

Sue: *'My father is dead but I have to be careful how and what I tell my mother about my symptoms in case it worries her.'*

Just because you now have MS doesn't mean that you can expect to resolve any or all such long-standing complications. There are those who find that the impact of an MS diagnosis is so profound as to trigger a realignment of all their closest relationships. In the process of redefining themselves and their future, they are able to break old emotional habits – for example, to give up trying either to please or to defy parents. For many others – probably the majority – adjusting the relationship with parents in the light of changed circumstances is just another aspect of coming to terms with MS. Given sufficient time and goodwill, you may be able to work out some kind of fit between what help and support your parents are willing and able to give and what you would like from them. Many people do achieve this successfully, but sadly a few find that parents (and sometimes in-laws too) have to be firmly discouraged from too much interference or over-protection.

> **Lizzy**: *'My mother originally suggested I move in with her, but having been to boarding school since I was eight, I have never really lived at home and could not contemplate it now. We get on very well in small doses, and I would hate to ruin it. This decision was the right one, as when she is with me she wants to do everything for me, and I believe in "use it or lose it". Had I lived with her, my MS would now be far worse.'*

> **Sarah**: *'My family panic when I talk about MS so I tend to keep quiet about it. I have an uncle with MS who is in his sixties but struggles to get about and be mobile. I think that because I look fine and "normal", they think I am OK, but I know what symptoms I will have "this week" and I'm the one who worries about them privately.'*

Friends

You may think you know someone really well, yet be unable to predict how they will respond to the fact of your MS. The good news is that you're likely to discover hidden depths in some of your friends and find that they are prepared to give more than you might have thought possible. Unfortunately, it's likely that you will also be in for some disappointments. Some people simply turn away from illness or disability of any kind – a reaction which has very little to do with you but is rooted in their own psyches. There are many possible explanations, such as an inability to face or share someone else's pain, a fear that you will demand more than they want or are prepared to give, or even the feeling that your misfortune is somehow contagious. There may even be an element of guilt or embarrassment that they are OK when you aren't. Whatever it is, you will find such people steering clear of you and there may be nothing you can do about it. Sometimes, good friends may draw back for fear of intruding or because they don't know what it is that you want from them. Much the same thing happens to the newly bereaved when people keep away or don't phone because they don't know what to say or do. You will probably have to make the first move making it clear that you would like to see someone and even bringing up the subject of MS so they know it's all right to talk about it.

Jenny: *'When I was first diagnosed, I found I was the one trying to cheer my friends up, seeing the funny side of MS and arranging visits and trips out. You just can't let yourself moan to some people because they get so upset on your behalf and you end up feeling worse than ever.'*

Sarah: *'I haven't told my friends – I don't want their sympathy but I also don't want them to think I'm a hypochondriac.'*

Frances: *'I find that some of my friends – that is, some of those who don't have MS – can be a bit over-protective at times.'*

Martin: *'My friends seem to pay little attention to my MS, which is just how I like it. But I feel that very few people understand the difficulties I face in everyday life – so many of my problems are not readily visible. However, one of the things I need most is friends who will help me through the dark days, and in this respect I'm lucky.'*

Experience will soon teach you which of your friends you can rely on when you need them. You'll probably turn to different people at different times as you always did – most of us have a range of friends who suit our different moods and different aspects of our personalities. Some friends may be useless when it comes to practical help, but just right when you need a laugh or a good gossip. Others will happily offer lifts or push the wheelchair, but are no good when you feel in need of some emotional support. And for much of the time, you may just want to enjoy whatever you did before, making as few concessions as possible to your MS. Perhaps you may be doing a bit less giving and a bit more accepting than you once did, but you'll want your friendships to remain on a more or less equal basis. You'd do well to be wary of the 'do-gooder' who starts being nice to you out of sympathy and who defines you primarily in terms of MS. That kind of 'friendship' may meet their needs, but doesn't have much to offer you.

Valerie: *'As a "people person", I would never have believed how many people find your illness more difficult than you do yourself. Hence many vanish or slowly withdraw through their own fears. After I had had to leave work because of my MS, one of my best friends phoned, very embarrassed, to tell me she had been given my old job. I was delighted – glad that someone I knew and liked had got it, and said so, but I never heard from her again. On the other hand, I've found new people have come forward, saying they'd always wanted to be friends, which has been great. There was one, however, who I eventually realized was simply using me because she was completely friendless herself. It took me about a year to realize that she wasn't what she seemed and not a true friend at all.'*

By the same token, there may be times when you have to ask yourself whether you are making demands on those close to you which they simply can't handle. When you are coping with major problems of your own, you can sometimes lose sight of the fact that your friends may have their own pressures. Paradoxically, they may feel guilty about mentioning them to you, still less complaining. After all, what are their problems compared to yours? Nevertheless, they're real enough and you may sometimes have to make an effort to acknowledge this. Of course, you may be perfectly willing to offer support and sympathy as you always have, but your friends stop expecting it of you. If you notice this is happening, it may be worth bringing the problem into the open, making it clear that you don't want to be excluded in this way. Even the most well-intentioned friends will get it wrong sometimes and you can begin to feel that you are living in a different universe from able-bodied people. Some people find that the only time they can let rip and say how they really feel is with other people who have MS. In a group where everyone knows at first hand how patronizing other people can be, what MS fatigue really feels like and has experienced the frustrations engendered by unpredictable symptoms, there's no need for politeness or pretence. This kind of get-together isn't for everyone, but if it does appeal, you'll find more on how to contact a local group on page 168.

Colleagues

Whether and when to tell people at work that you have MS can present a real dilemma. There are several good reasons why you might choose to keep your diagnosis to yourself. The first is simply to protect your privacy. You may also be concerned about the reaction of colleagues – both on a personal basis and in terms of its effect on your future prospects. In any case, there may be no reason for anyone to know if your symptoms are minor and have no impact on your ability to do your job. So much depends on how you are affected and what skills or abilities are vital to your performance at work. A physically demanding job may well mean having no choice about acknowledging your difficulties at a relatively early stage.

> **Frances**: *'I was a nurse when I was first diagnosed in 1988, and had worked full-time. I was able to carry on part-time for about 18 months, but then I had to retire when the symptoms got worse. I tire very easily and can't move about very well and sometimes my balance is affected.'*

However, if you are able to continue working, you may well go through periods when symptoms worsen and are more difficult to hide. What's more, concealment means you can't ask for understanding or any kind of support and the mental strain of keeping your secret is an extra burden.

> **Chloe:** *'For the moment I've not told my employers about my condition. I've thought very hard about the ethics, advantages and disadvantages. I think there are many misconceptions about the disease (partly perpetuated by past MS Society campaigns unfortunately), such as assuming that all people with MS lose their eyesight and are permanently wheelchair-bound. I know for a fact that my colleagues and bosses at work have these prejudices and am concerned that they would treat me differently if they knew I had the disease. I'm sure that it would jeopardize any chance of my promotion with my present company. The industry I work in is quite insular and I'm concerned MS would count against me with prospective employers too.'*

However well-founded fears like these may be, there may be no avoiding the issue in the end. Either the symptoms may worsen so that your ill-health becomes obvious to everyone or you may find the pretence impossible to sustain indefinitely. Even when it's possible to continue working with the appearance of normality, many people find their MS exacts a very high price. Evenings and weekends are devoted to recovering from the stresses of the working day, so there's virtually no energy left for other areas of life.

When you do decide to tell people at work, it's a good idea to follow it up with some facts about MS and the way it is affecting you. Unless they are unusually well-informed, most people are likely to know little about the symptoms of MS or what the consequences might be for you or for them. It will probably help if you can explain in what ways you are unlikely to be affected as well; as Chloe pointed out, to most people MS implies severe handicap and probably rapid decline into death. This may also be the best time to ask for any organizational or practical changes which will help you to fulfil the demands of your job. For example, you may be able to station yourself somewhere which is handy for the loo, or doesn't require you to climb stairs or to sit on top of a radiator. No one will think of these things unless you suggest them, but colleagues and bosses may be happy to co-operate once they know what you need. Don't forget to mention any 'invisible' symptoms either – especially fatigue. Having an 'official' rest at lunch-time could make all the difference some days if fatigue is a particular problem for you. You may also think it worth trying to negotiate flexible working hours which allow you to travel in greater comfort at times when public transport is less crowded.

Once everyone realizes that you can still function effectively despite having MS, the advantages of being open about your condition may outweigh the disadvantages. This isn't always the case, however. There are companies which take a completely negative view of any health problem, refuse to adapt in any way and even make efforts to get rid of you. You may become a prime target for dismissal or redundancy or just put under pressure to go voluntarily. Anyone who knows or suspects this may be happening should make sure they check out their legal position, and enlist the support of a professional organization, trade union or personnel officer if at all possible. For more on this, see pages 142–3.

More subtle discrimination can be almost as hard to deal with. Even when you are certain you're being denied promotion or the chance to rise to an interesting challenge, you may be able to do little or nothing about it. Your superiors may not even be discriminating consciously or they may feel that your condition genuinely precludes you from moving up the promotion ladder. It may be worth tackling the question head-on if you think you can convince the relevant people that they are mistaken. It also has to be said that in some instances they could be right. If you are inclined to underestimate the effect of your MS symptoms or the demands a particular job would put on you, you may be forced to accept that your bosses have made the correct decision from their point of view.

Robin: *'I had to retire early from my job as a qualified electrical engineer because of my MS four years ago. Now I do voluntary playwork to help disabled children. I'm still happy to push myself to the limits, but I can only do it part-time. Helping the children helps me, and I like to be involved. I now feel that 'life is what you make it'. I once worked as an engineer on shift in power stations and writing major reports. Now perhaps I might give my time and effort instead to help a group of children or even just one child – which is the more important?'*

Sue: *'At first I reduced the hours I worked in my job, then eventually I stopped altogether. Struggling with the demands of a career and the demands of MS left work undone – I felt guilty and as if I were being carried by my colleagues – and left no time for me. Now I have my life back, albeit a changed life, but then life is changing anyway. Now I do voluntary work, about eight hours a week for the Citizens Advice Bureau which keeps the brain* *on-line and makes me feel useful. When I was still working in my career, I was resting at lunchtime, then going straight to bed when I got home. Weekends were spent doing nothing but recharging an increasingly faulty battery. The result was no quality of life.'*

7

FINDING A PATTERN

A person with MS has no choice but to live with the condition in the best way they can. In practical terms, you're unlikely to be able to carry on living as though nothing has changed even though you now have the diagnosis. When symptoms are minor or you have long periods of remission, it may seem as if things are going on much as before. Even so, there is now an element of uncertainty about the future which is bound to have an impact on your life. More significant symptoms or an illness which appears to be progressive with little or no respite will take a more obvious and immediate toll.

The adjustments you have to make in your life may be small or large, and there may be quite long periods when things seem to be on a relatively even keel. Some people prefer to postpone getting any kind of help – be it emotional, practical, medical or financial – until the need arises. Others plan ahead so that everything is in place if or when circumstances change. What follows in this section is a digest of information which you can choose to make use of as and when you need to. Probably no one person will need all of it.

Someone who's naturally self-reliant may deeply dislike

135

the idea of applying for benefits or even a special orange badge to claim parking privileges. Having your home or car modified or resorting to wheelchair or walking stick is a recognition that you are affected by MS and so may be something you resist bitterly. It is nevertheless a fact that by acknowledging that you could benefit from the right kind of help at the right time, you can make it possible to circumvent some of the limitations which MS would otherwise impose on your lifestyle. If you are able to accept this realistically, you can fight the battle against the condition in a way which makes some kind of victory achievable. While you can't do anything to make MS go away, you can often take steps to make it more manageable.

As part of the process of learning to live with your MS, you may find you need to reassess your priorities. For example, someone who's prone to fatigue may have to accept that burning the candle at both ends is no longer an option. You may conclude that there are some things that you can cut out without really missing them to give yourself more energy for the things that really matter to you. An overcrowded schedule can leave you exhausted and stressed so that you can't really enjoy anything properly. Reassessing your priorities and cutting out unnecessary clutter can ease the pressure with positive results in terms of your health and general well-being.

Symptom triggers

Although MS can always spring surprises, you may learn to recognize certain patterns or recurring features of your own disease. As ever, some will be unique to you, others familiar to many other people with MS. You might also like to keep at the back of your mind that having MS doesn't make you immune from other conditions. In other words, don't always assume automatically that a new symptom must be related to MS: it could possibly have another – treatable – cause.

Most people find that there are certain things which can trigger a worsening of their symptoms. This doesn't necessarily mean that the MS has changed, but that you become more aware of existing symptoms. Brief periods when you experience a temporary change for the worse are usually called exacerbations and may last minutes or days. A relapse normally involves one or more new symptoms or the reappearance of old ones, and can last for months.

Many people with MS say that a relapse does not come out of the blue. Although they sometimes only recognize it after the event, they experience some change which affects them psychologically. Some talk of becoming more emotionally volatile – veering suddenly from laughter to tears, others of increased irritability or a lack of mental flexibility. Sometimes it seems that it's hard to think at all and the person has a sense of losing control of what's happening. You may not recognize this phase as part of your experience, or if you do, you may want to express it quite differently. For those who have this kind of advance warning, there may be the opportunity to ease off a little and possibly shorten the duration of the relapse or limit its severity. At the very least, you may feel better prepared to face it and deal with the consequences.

Fatigue

Fatigue is one of the commonest features of MS, and it's especially significant because it frequently brings other problems in its wake. For many people, it is a prime symptom in itself. As you will know if you've experienced it, it can come on fast and apparently unprovoked and is completely irresistible. With normal tiredness, you can sometimes get a second wind in the right circumstances, and then keep going for hours after you first started to droop. There's no question of this with fatigue and you just have to rest. When it happens a lot, you may have no choice but to rearrange your life to allow for it.

It's enough of a nuisance on its own, but for many people, fatigue is often accompanied by a change in other symptoms. An old symptom which you thought had disappeared may come back or an existing one become more noticeable or severe. Sometimes, you may get a symptom that's new to you but which only lasts as long as the fatigue.

It's not clear why this fatigue occurs, but it's likely that the nerve impulses are considerably weaker than normal because demyelination means they have to struggle to reach their destination. This might explain not only the fatigue, but the other symptoms which can accompany it, depending on which nerves are involved. So your limbs may feel heavy and sluggish, your vision become a bit fuzzy or you may find it a real effort to formulate and express thoughts and ideas. All these or other peculiar symptoms mean that the relevant nerves are not performing normally. If you can identify some kind of pattern in the onset of fatigue you may be able to reduce its severity and duration, even though you can't avoid it altogether.

Timing is crucial for some people – with the late afternoon being when they're most likely to find their energy dipping. It's been suggested that this may be connected to the fact that body temperature reaches its daily peak around this time of day. This makes sense in view of the fact that heat triggers fatigue and many other symptoms for a lot of people with MS. In particular, a hot bath can sometimes produce dramatic effects. As well as fatigue, it can bring on 'new' symptoms and make old ones worse. The reason for this seems to be that increasing the body temperature somehow brings into the open the effects of myelin damage which are not normally apparent. This can become evident in two ways: you could actually experience the effects of the neurological damage yourself, and a neurologist could detect it by checking reflexes and other signs. Neither signs nor symptoms would normally show up, and they will gradually disappear again once your temperature returns to normal.

If you do react to overheating in this way, you'll probably find it happens after you've been exerting yourself or when you have an infection as well as after a hot bath. Hot weather is obviously going to be no fun for you, especially as air conditioning is still relatively rare in the UK. Some people have found it helps to wear special 'cool suits' – waistcoats containing coolant liquid. You may be able to find them for sale second-hand through the MS Resource Centre's newsletter *Pathways* (see page 151) and they can also provide details of suppliers. For details of a new, cheaper model contact Midicool 01252 372466.

Although excessive heat is a more common trigger, there are some people for whom cold is the problem and there are other culprits too. You may be one of those who find that fatigue comes on after a heavy meal, and smoking often makes the problem worse. Some of these triggers are easier to avoid than others, and sometimes your options will be limited. You can do nothing about hot weather, for example, although an electric fan and regular cool showers or baths may help a bit. In winter, you may be able to negotiate with those who share your living and/or working space to keep heating at a tolerable level or to have your nearest radiator turned down or off.

> **Lizzy:** *'I find I'm worse when it's cold as well as when it's hot. In the winter, I go out as little as possible. I've got an area in my lounge which stays pretty cool, so I keep in there when it's really hot.'*

Despite your best efforts, fatigue is likely to get you from time to time, and then rest is your only option. This is particularly frustrating if you've always been an energetic person, packing the maximum activity into every twenty-four hours. When your body won't allow you to do all the things you want to, you have no choice but to adapt. Some people who have been compelled to do this have said afterwards that it brought them gains as well as losses. Not being able to do everything can provide the incentive to think about what really matters and set new priorities.

> **Helena:** *'My counsellor suggested I make a list of all the things I could still do and enjoy, and those I couldn't. I was sad that I couldn't run any more, for instance, but I was surprised at how many things there were on the positive list. That helped me to start looking forward rather than concentrating on what I'd lost.'*

> **Sue:** *'I've stopped my physical activities and now do more sedentary-type things – which I enjoy. For example, I've bought a computer and this has opened a whole new world*

and I've become involved in the disability movement. I now have less free time outside my rest periods than I used to.'

Frequent strenuous exercise may have to be abandoned – either because you can't physically do it any more or because your body takes ever longer to recover afterwards. However, even if you can't continue playing squash or running marathons, you may be able to carry on swimming, dancing or exercise classes, for example. It depends on how your MS affects you and you may be able to do more at some periods than others. The point is not to overdo it so that you knock yourself out and have to spend days recuperating afterwards. The same is true of other aspects of your life. You can develop a 'feel' for what is reasonable and what isn't in terms of its effect on your MS. Of course there are likely to be times when you do the unreasonable anyway, either because of circumstances or just because you feel like it. You may accept that you'll simply have to pay the price in terms of fatigue afterwards on this occasion. However, if you push yourself to the limit too often you may end up feeling quite ill as a result.

Stress

It's become something of a habit with most of us to blame stress for causing just about everything from the common cold to road rage. Similarly, many people believe it is responsible for making their MS symptoms worse or bringing on a relapse. In fact, stress does not entirely deserve its bad press. Most of us need a certain amount of it to galvanize us into doing things we would otherwise put off. One person's stress is another's incentive, and some people positively thrive on it. Up to a point, it's a question of how we respond and that's very much an individual thing. Trouble comes when we feel overwhelmed by it so that we can't function properly.

Psychologists have looked at life events which seem to be associated with increased stress and are likely to produce adverse effects. Interestingly, it's not just the obvious things like a bereavement or divorce which come high on the list, but also positive experiences like holidays and getting married. Our bodies react to severe stress by producing specialized hormones, designed by evolution to help cope with the expected crisis. This was fine for primitive man who was then better equipped to tackle a predator or run for his life, but less use today when emergencies are usually of a different order. We don't burn off stress hormones through physical activity, and if the stressful situation isn't resolved the hormones continue to circulate. We feel tense and anxious and our body chemistry is out of balance which can reduce the efficiency of the immune system.

Precisely how all this affects the symptoms of MS isn't clear. Prolonged stress which leaves you constantly on edge and interferes with your ability to eat and sleep will increase your fatigue and so may make other symptoms worse. Whether stress can actually provoke a relapse is open to debate, but in any case the answer is likely to depend on the nature of the stress and how you personally react to it. It's clear enough that stress which makes you feel bad or interferes with your mental or physical functioning is no good for your health either. Many people with MS have learned that their symptoms do get worse during or after periods of major stress.

Lizzy: *'Stress is probably the most influential factor in my MS, particularly when I feel it is aimed at me personally or threatens me financially. This is why I always say it was unemployment which triggered my MS. No one should be expected to live on unemployment benefit and survive, particularly not in a recession and when new technology means less jobs.'*

Chloe: *'I have found that all of my significant attacks have been stress-related. The first was a couple of months after my finals exams at university; then I lost the use of my hand after a particularly stressful time at work and a recent exacerbation followed on from an emotionally traumatic time in my life.'*

Sarah: *'I can link each attack with a stressful time in my life. The first, when I was twelve, with starting secondary school; aged fifteen with studying for exams; twenty-one, starting a new job and twenty-seven, moving house with a new baby.'*

At what might be called the micro level, certain kinds of stress can have an unmistakable effect. For example, if you can't walk very well, being put under pressure can slow you down more than usual. Trying to get to the front door before the caller gives up and leaves is guaranteed to make many people with MS feel they're wearing lead boots. Some say that a major row or other emotional drama has a similar effect, but the consequences in terms of symptom-worsening are generally short-lived. It may have something to do with panic or emotional arousal causing your temperature to rise, but anyway it isn't permanent. You may need to remind yourself – or those close to you – of this sometimes. When there seems to be a link between this sort of stressful situation and a worsening of MS symptoms, people can start going to all kinds of lengths to avoid provoking any stress. They may start treating you like some delicate flower that must be shielded from anything potentially upsetting. Sometimes, too, a person with MS can be tempted to exploit the situation for their own ends. A sort of moral blackmail develops in which they use the threat of being made worse to get their own way and control other people.

When stress is used in either of these ways, it can end up putting unnecessary limitations on the way you live your life. Rather than try to exclude all stress you might do better finding ways of coping with it. There are both psychological and practical approaches to the problem. For example, you could deal with the impatient visitor at the front door in several ways: resolve to let them wait, install an entryphone or put up a notice asking callers to be patient. Learning to deal calmly with potentially stressful situations isn't particularly easy for most people but it is worth trying. Some people find relaxation or meditation classes or tapes are a help, and yoga enables many of its practitioners to respond better to stress.

Minor illnesses

One of the ironies of MS is that many people who have it say they hardly ever suffer from minor illnesses like colds and flu. It's hard to imagine why this might be so, but such infections can certainly have repercussions and may trigger a relapse. While you have the infection and for some time afterwards, you may be troubled with new and possibly alarming symptoms. Some people find they disappear quickly, but they may continue for weeks before fading or never disappear altogether.

Jenny: *'I had a nasty dose of flu, but as it started to pass I found my eyesight was affected for the first time ever. I had blurred and sometimes double vision, and I couldn't talk or eat properly because one side of my face felt like it was paralysed. It was much worse than any other of my MS symptoms and I was very frightened. My doctor prescribed my first course of steroid tablets, and the symptoms gradually disappeared over the next few weeks. That was two years ago, and although I'm much less mobile now, I can see normally and move my face which for me is much more important.'*

Pregnancy

The chances are greater today that someone with MS will be diagnosed at an age when they have not yet taken on parenthood. Of course, there are still some people who don't find out that they have the condition until after they've had a family, but this is less common than in earlier generations. Many people will be glad they are in a position to take MS into account when planning whether and when to have children. However, it also makes the decision harder for most couples. As well as considering the impact on their own lives, couples worry whether the MS might be passed on to their children. Although it is not genetically transmitted in any straightforward way, a child born to a parent with MS does have a higher than normal risk of developing it. Experts estimate the risk to be 1–3 in 100.

The decision is most difficult when it's the woman who

has MS. The major worry is whether a pregnancy would make her MS worse, and how her body will cope with the stress of delivery and its after effects. The potential problems are not as obvious when it's the man who has MS, but he and his partner may still be concerned about what the future holds in terms of his health. Will his MS symptoms interfere with his ability to be the kind of father he wants to be, for example? It may be important that he continues to be able to support the family financially if his partner plans to be a full-time mother. There's also the question of the demands a young child makes on parents' time and energy, which may be more of a strain when one partner has MS.

It may be easier if you know you can rely on family and friends nearby to share the workload or if you can afford to pay for any help you need. Even so, you need to consider the long term too: teenagers can be at least as demanding and exhausting in their own way as babies and toddlers.

These are issues which each couple will think through for themselves. However, it is worth bearing in mind that no one can rely on good health or a guaranteed income when they decide to have children, even though they may not have MS to contend with. If would-be parents only considered the potential difficulties, very few would ever have children at all!

Pregnancy is a demanding and complicated business physically speaking and it does make sense to consider the effect it will have on you when you have MS. At one time, women with MS were often advised against getting pregnant, but this is much less likely today unless a woman has severe disabilities. If you've recently had a bad relapse, it's generally a good idea to wait at least a year before getting pregnant. The ideal is probably to leave it until you've gone two years without a serious relapse. The trouble with this advice, however, is that you don't know how long it will take you to conceive. As a general rule, the older you are, the longer it is likely to take you, but there are plenty of exceptions. MS does not affect fertility, but many normally fertile couples find it takes months or longer for the woman to conceive. For others, it's virtually instant, so planning the best time theoretically for you to be pregnant doesn't necessarily work out in practice.

> **Jenny**: *'Although I now believe I had my first MS symptoms at nineteen, they weren't recognized as such. If I'd known that I had MS, I definitely would have thought twice about having a family. In fact, both my pregnancies were trouble-free and my symptoms have only become a problem in the last few years. My two daughters are now teenagers, and I would have hated to miss out on being a mum.'*

It is sensible to talk over your plans with your GP or neurologist. Hopefully they will know you and your MS well and can discuss any potential problems in the light of your personal experience. In any case, you need to ask about any drugs which you are taking on a regular basis in case it's advisable to change or stop them in pregnancy. You might also have to consider whether your MS symptoms are likely to cause any specific problems, either with pregnancy or delivery. For example, balance and mobility problems, as well as fatigue, may get worse, especially towards the end of pregnancy when most women feel tired in any case. A normal labour may not be possible if your muscle tone is affected, and you may not have the option of an epidural anaesthetic if you experience any numbness.

It's not all bad news, however. Many women with MS feel quite well in pregnancy, especially in the middle three months. It's important to look after your general health, making sure you eat well and get plenty of sleep. If you're normally a very busy person, pregnancy may give you an incentive to slow down and rest when you need to.

Towards the end of your pregnancy, you will want to consider the kind of birth you will have. You may be able to discuss your pain relief options with the anaesthetist in advance, and your midwife and obstetrician should help you to plan the delivery you want, taking into account any possible physical limitations.

It is once your baby is born that you are most at risk of suffering a relapse – with around one in five women affected in the first few months. No one knows quite why this should be, although prime suspects include hormonal changes and the demands of caring for a new baby. It's wise to prepare as much as you can, especially by arranging for as much practical help as possible to be available. It might mean your partner or a relative taking over domestically or arranging for a home help. Your energy needs to be conserved so that you can care for your baby and for your own well-being. It is especially important to do whatever you can to avoid getting too tired or putting yourself under any other kind of pressure. Sometimes this may mean bottle-feeding rather than breast-feeding your baby which can be physically draining for a new mother. If you were keen to breast-feed but find it is too much for you, you're bound to be disappointed. Try not to let it get to you and to accept that you're doing the best thing for yourself and your baby.

Even though there is an increased chance of a relapse after having a baby, you may still be one of the majority of new mothers whose MS stays much the same. Either way, it could be an opportune moment to consult an occupational therapist about any gadgets or modifications which could be made to your home to make life easier. Even if you've resisted the idea before, you need all your energy and strength from now on, so it's worth taking advantage of anything that helps to conserve them.

Contact with other women in the neighbourhood is a lifeline for many new mothers, especially when they don't have friends or family nearby. Being able to compare notes and share experiences can boost your confidence because you realize that others are finding it just as hard to cope with a crying baby or broken nights, even though they don't have MS!

Because relapses can follow pregnancy, people once tended to assume that the two were cause and effect. In fact, pregnancy and childbirth don't appear to have any long-term effect on the progress of MS. Research has shown that after ten years, the condition had not led to greater disability in mothers than in women who had not had children.

Surgery and anaesthetics

Although there have been reports that surgery and/or anaesthetics can trigger an exacerbation of MS, the evidence is what doctors call 'anecdotal'. In other words, there is no real medical evidence to support these stories which are based on individual experience. The unpredictability of MS means that, without proper controlled trials (which have not been done), it's impossible to say that a relapse which follows an operation was caused by it – it might well have happened anyway.

chapter eight

PRACTICAL AND FINANCIAL HELP

There are many reasons why you may be reluctant to ask for or accept any of the various types of help to which you could be entitled. For many people with MS, using a stick or applying for an orange badge implies that they are 'giving in' or changing into a different kind of person – one who is defined by the condition or by his or her disabilities. What's more, for some this seems like a double admission: not only are you acknowledging that you can't stand on your own two feet literally, but also that you can't do so metaphorically either. In other words, the idea of accepting help in the form of benefits or special services goes against the grain of independence and self-sufficiency. This is hard, but there are other ways of looking at it. For example, you could regard the various aids available as tools to enable you to go on living the kind of life you want. Used appropriately, a stick or a wheelchair may make it possible for you to get to places and do things you otherwise couldn't; modifications to your home may mean you can go on living independently. By applying for benefits to which you are entitled because of your MS, you are not taking charity but simply using your rights in the same way other people do when they send their children to state schools or get free contraceptives on prescription!

> **Sue:** *'I was chatting with an elderly relative who has difficulty walking and suggested that she try using a stick occasionally, but no, she's independent and stubborn (I wonder if it runs in the family?). It reminded me of the time when I first had difficulties with mobility, and I wouldn't use anything, apart from walls and furniture, to steady myself. It was silly I suppose, but I didn't want to seem disabled and I wasn't elderly, so I didn't need a stick to walk. Then I gave it a try – with a stylish black folding stick. Suddenly, I found it helped me to balance, gave me that bit of support when I needed it, warned strangers not to bump into me and I could use it to reach things on the floor: I could even use it to hit people I didn't like – well, not literally, but you know the feeling . . .'*

Health and social services

Responsibility for providing help in the form of services, aids and information to make life easier is shared between local authority social services departments and the NHS. This may cover anything from a walking stick to help with shopping, depending on your requirements. What's available will also vary depending on where you live as individual social services departments don't all interpret their responsibilities in precisely the same way. The details of the NHS and Community Care Act 1990, which lays out duties and provisions, are complex and in some cases the practical applications are still being worked out. For full details of the current state of play, you may like to read the MS Society's information sheets on Community Care.

MOBILITY

As you will already be in contact with your GP, he or she may be able to guide you towards the various people you can call on for help and advice. For example, they can arrange for you to have walking sticks or other mobility aids. Wheelchairs are actually provided via social services, but your GP or hospital doctor will have to complete an application form on your behalf.

Recent changes mean that as well as hand-controlled wheelchairs, the NHS can now also supply powered ones for use outside as well as indoors for people with severe disabilities. The Department of Health is in the process of introducing a new wheelchair voucher scheme with the aim of giving users more choice. Rather than simply accepting a standard NHS model, individuals could opt for an assessment of their needs, and could then be allocated vouchers equivalent to the cost of the wheelchair which the NHS would have supplied and use them to contribute to the cost of a more sophisticated model. The plan is to phase the scheme in over a number of years, and further information will be available in due course from GPs, health centres and physiotherapy and occupational therapy departments in each area. Alternatively, you may be able to buy a wheelchair on an HP basis through the Motability scheme if you receive the higher rate mobility component of the Disability Living Allowance. Details of how the scheme operates with respect to wheelchairs, powered scooters and cars can be obtained from: Motability, Goodman House, Station Approach, Harlow, Essex CM20 2ET; tel: 01279 635666.

Do shop around and try wheelchairs for yourself before making a decision; an occupational therapist will be able to tell you how and where you can do this.

Wheelchairs and other means of getting around have a symbolic significance both for people with disabilities and for many of the rest of the population too. Many people feel, with justification, that using one has a profoundly detrimental effect on their sense of self and predisposes other people to look down on them, metaphorically as well as literally. It's not an easy dilemma to resolve. Increased mobility and independence have to be weighed against the psychological and social disadvantages. Many people opt for a compromise – using one when the situation leaves little alternative, while refusing to let it become a habit.

Janet: *'In general, I work on the principle that anything I can't do on my feet I don't want to do at all. However, I did use a wheelchair recently when I was going on holiday otherwise I'd never have made it along the miles of airport corridor to get to the plane.'*

Lizzy: *'I have a manual wheelchair on the NHS but I would love an electric one. I'm someone who's always in too much of a hurry – I used to run and skip rather than walk, so an electric wheelchair would speed me up. I can only use the manual one if someone pushes me. The only time I tried wheeling it myself for a few feet, I couldn't lift a saucepan for ages afterwards. I don't mind going out in it, but I won't use it indoors if I can avoid it because I don't want to become totally dependent on it.'*

Hazel: *'Since I've had to stop driving our car, I have been able to get a small Batricar so I can now get to the shops and back, which is great.'*

Before buying any kind of vehicle or having your own car adapted, it is worth getting proper advice on what would suit you best. One of the best sources of practical help are the various driver assessment centres around the country. They do charge – usually around £100 – but if having your needs properly assessed means you avoid expensive mistakes, it is money well spent. You can also get information from the Department of Transport Mobility Advice and Vehicle Information Centre, TRL, Crowthorne, Berkshire RG45 6AU. Information is free, but you will have to pay for detailed advice. It's also worth contacting the Mobility Information Service, who can send leaflets giving guidance on getting the right car for your needs. Contact them at Unit 2A, Atcham Industrial Estate, Upton Magna, Shrewsbury SY4 4UG; tel: 01743 761889.

Even if you're an experienced driver, driving a specially adapted car takes some getting used to and many people find it helps to take a short course of lessons to build up their confidence. A number of driving schools, including BSM, can arrange this, using either your own vehicle or their own suitably adapted ones. BSM now has over 150 instructors who have received special training at the Banstead Mobility Centre and you can contact the BSM Central Mobility Unit on 0181 540 8262. A list of assessment centres, including some with adapted cars and specialist instructors, is available from the Disabled Drivers Association. Contact them on 01508 489449. They also have useful leaflets, including a general one on mobility called *Sorry I'm Late Again!*, and can answer specific queries by letter and phone.

Lizzy: *'I got a car through Motability and I've recently had it adapted. They've put a removable false floor in front of the driving seat because the brake pedal was too high. It can be* *taken out if someone else is driving. So far, I'm only doing short journeys, but it's much easier to drive now.'*

You will obviously need insurance if you do have a car, and it's a good idea to have a wheelchair insured as well. For information on companies which can arrange this, contact the MS Society for their leaflet *Insurance and MS*. The Motability brochure includes a list of suitable insurance companies. You might also like to join the Disabled Drivers Association, who have a list of companies who can arrange insurance for their members. You will also need to let the DVLA know that you have MS; contact the Medical Advisory Branch, Dept of Transport, Oldway Centre, Orchard Street, Swansea SA99 1TU; tel: 01792 783438.

If you do have a car, whether adapted or not, you should enquire about whether you are entitled to an orange badge which will free you from many of the normal parking restrictions and entitle you to make use of reserved parking spaces. Contact your local social services department for details of how to apply.

HELP AT HOME

When it comes to aids and gadgets for the home, you'll find it useful to get expert help because the range on offer is enormous. Occupational therapists, who work either in hospitals or for the local social services department, are the people you need to contact. They can visit you in your home and discuss what you need, explain what's available and how to obtain what you want. It may be something relatively minor that will make all the difference – such as a handrail or a ramp which you need to have installed at home or other aids which will make things like bathing easier and safer. You can also get advice and information on what's available from The Disabled Living Foundation, 380-4 Harrow Road, London W9 2HU; tel: 0171 289 6111. They can tell you how to contact your nearest 'Aids to Daily Living' Centre where you can see a range of aids and gadgets (including wheelchairs and scooters) and get expert advice from occupational therapists and physiotherapists. Other services are available through the social services department, including personal care, or sometimes domestic help with things like housework or shopping, concessions on public transport and access to day centres. You may not want all or any of these at the moment, but it's useful to be aware of the possibilities in case your circumstances change.

> **Lizzy:** *'Having my house adapted has made a big difference. I discussed what was to be done with the occupational therapist, and I only had to pay for extras like tiling because I'm on income support. I've got a new kitchen and a lift, and downstairs I now have a loo and shower room, which is a brilliant bonus. Unfortunately, I now need the front entrance adapted because I can't get down the steps and the council said it should have been done at the same time as the other work. However, I'm fighting the decision and my occupational therapist has gone back to them and we are hoping they will change their mind.'*

A social worker or occupational therapist may suggest that you register with social services as someone whose disability is 'substantial or permanent' or they may register you automatically when you contact them. This will ensure that you receive information on what is available, and even if you don't need anything specific at the moment, being registered may help those in charge when planning their services to meet the needs of people with disabilities.

As part of the policy of community care, local health authorities provide a number of community health services designed to help people remain at home as far as possible instead of being admitted to hospital. If necessary, your GP can arrange for you to have regular home visits from the district (or community) nurse, who can help with bathing or dressing as well as providing actual nursing care and help with continence problems. She or he can also put you in touch with a specialist continence advisor who can discuss with you what medications or aids are available to meet your needs. Alternatively, you can phone the Continence Foundation's Helpline on 0191 213 0050 to contact your local advisor. The nurse or advisor will also know whether there is a laundry service in your area and how to arrange for disposal of incontinence pads or dressings. They can also help to arrange for you to have a commode at home if this would be useful. In some circumstances, grants may be available through the DSS towards the cost of having an extra downstairs loo built in your house – talk to a social worker about whether you could be eligible.

The MS Society publishes a detailed and very useful guide called *Be Continent, Be Confident*, which explains more about the various forms of equipment and other help available. They also have a fund which can make grants to help pay for alterations to your home or other necessities. Applications have to be made through a local branch in the first instance; in practice some may prefer to give priority to branch members although anyone with MS can apply.

BENEFITS

Working out which benefits you may be entitled to, obtaining and completing the necessary forms can be daunting to say the least. It is hardly surprising that many people are not receiving everything they should, but there is help available from various organizations. The official source of information for the majority of benefits is The Benefits Agency who publish a stack of free leaflets available from any post office or social security office. Alternatively, they are available by post from BA Distribution and Storage Centre, Heywood Stores, Manchester Road, Heywood, Lancs OL10 2PZ. When in doubt, start with *A Guide to Benefits* (FB2) and *Which Benefit* (BG1). There is a free Benefits Enquiry Line on 0800 882200 or Welsh Benefits Enquiry Line 0800 289011 (Monday to Friday 10 a.m. to 10 p.m.). You can also get advice from your local social security office whose number is in the phone book. It is important to get in touch without delay if you think you may not be claiming a benefit to which you're entitled otherwise you could lose out financially. For detailed guidance on benefits and how to claim, the *Disability Rights Handbook*, published annually by the Disability Alliance ERA, is invaluable. It costs £9.95; £5.95 for those claiming benefit. The Disability Alliance can also answer individual queries; ring them on 0171 247 8776.

Some benefits are targeted at those who are not in paid work or who have a low income; others are specifically for people with disabilities to cover some of the extra expense incurred because of physical or other limitations. In some cases, your entitlement will depend on NI contributions, including the new Incapacity Benefit for people under the age of sixty-five for men and sixty for women who cannot work due to illness or disability. This has replaced the old Sickness and Invalidity Benefits and your capacity for work will be assessed when you apply. The Benefits Agency has a special telephone helpline which you can ring for information leaflets on 0800 868868.

Other benefits, such as the Disability Living Allowance (DLA) and Disability Working Allowance (DWA), are not means-tested and do not depend on NI contributions.

Changes to Income Support are being introduced and Unemployment Benefit is being replaced by the new Jobseekers Allowance for people who are not exempted from signing on. Both are covered in the latest edition of the *Disability Rights Handbook*. Income Support is a particularly important benefit because if you are entitled to it, you may also be entitled to other linked benefits, such as housing and council tax benefits and free prescriptions and dental care. As well as your local social services department, advice and information is available from Citizens Advice Bureaux. The welfare officers at the MS Society can give you advice on how to get more information, and they also produce an excellent leaflet outlining all the benefits with details on how to make a claim. It's called *Social Security Benefits and MS* and is available free by post.

In the working world

For those who have jobs, MS may interfere early on with their ability to carry on doing them, depending on its severity or what particular abilities it affects. Others will be faced with deciding whether to tell employers and colleagues that they have MS. There are plenty of good reasons why many people choose to keep quiet. However, while you are not obliged to tell your employer that you have

MS, you do have a legal duty to let them know of any disability which could affect your safety at work or that of your colleagues.

You could put yourself in an awkward position if you conceal the fact that you have MS when applying for a new job. The employer could be within their rights to dismiss you when they found out, whereas you'd have a better chance of claiming unfair dismissal if they got rid of you because of your MS, even though they knew about it when you joined. There are various schemes and organizations which try to help people with disabilities find work. No one expects finding a new job to be easy these days so it's worth pursuing all possible avenues of help. At the Job Centres run by the Employment Service, you should be able to make contact with so-called PACT teams. PACT stands for Placing, Assessment and Counselling Teams, who specialize in giving advice on everything relating to the employment of people with disabilities. The Disability Employment Advisor (DEA) works with both employers and people seeking work, giving advice on recruitment and training, access, adaptations and equipment – including financial help towards the cost and specific schemes like Access to Work. They may also liaise between an employer and a person with disabilities under the Job Introduction Scheme, which offers financial assistance to allow someone to be employed for a trial period. This is intended to give both parties an opportunity to find out whether the person and the job suit each other.

Other organizations offering a job-finding service and advice on education and training for people with disabilities and potential employers include:

- Association of Disabled Professionals, 170 Benton Hill, Horbury, Wakefield WF4 5HW; tel: 01924 270335.

- Opportunities for People with Disabilities, I Bank
  Buildings, Princes Street, London EC2R 8EU; tel: 0171 726
  4961.

Travel and holidays

Companies in the travel and tourism business are slowly
waking up to the fact that they need to work harder to attract
custom from people with disabilities. Where those involved
have made a special effort to provide the necessary information and facilities, it's just a matter of making your choice
and booking in the usual way. Unless you are dealing with
specialists, however, you'd do well to take nothing on trust
unless you've checked it out yourself as much as you can.
This may involve ringing the tour operator or hotel personally and asking them specifically about any aspects that are
important to you. It's also worth following up any phone
conversations with a letter or fax confirming the arrangements in writing, especially for important details such as
ground floor accommodation. This is less of a problem in
this country, but if you're going abroad, time spent dotting
the i's and crossing the t's will be a good investment. You
may do better dealing with the smaller outfits when it comes
to tour operators or travel agents because they are more likely
to know the destination and the accommodation personally
and be able to answer your questions.

An invaluable source of information and advice, particularly for those planning a break in the UK, is a charity called
the Holiday Care Service. They keep comprehensive data on
travel, accommodation and tourist attractions and are happy

to try and answer any query you have by phone. For practical reasons, the information on foreign destinations is less detailed, but there are fact sheets available on around thirty countries, with sources of further information included. Other leaflets include *Holiday Centres (Caravans and Chalets)*, *Activity or Special Interest Holidays* and *Respite Care Stays (Residential or Nursing Homes)*. They also publish the useful *Holiday Care Guide to Accessible Travel*, which lists over 1,000 hotels, guest houses and self-catering establishments which have all been inspected for ease of access. Published annually, it costs £5.95 including postage and packing. For £10 a year, you can become a 'Friend of Holiday Care', which entitles you to a discount on the guide plus use of the organization's reservations service, a regular newsletter and details of special offers. Contact the Holiday Care Service at: 2nd Floor, Imperial Buildings, Victoria Road, Horley, Surrey RH6 7PZ; tel: 01293 774535.

When going abroad, it is vital to make sure you have a suitable insurance policy that covers all your requirements. Tour operators and travel agents are usually keen to sell you their policies at the time of booking, but these may not necessarily be the most suitable or the best value for money. Make sure that you read the small print and check specifically the provision for health care and arrangements for getting you home should the need arise. The MS Society's leaflet *Insurance and MS* suggests two companies who offer policies tailored for people with MS: Extrasure Holding Ltd, 6 Lloyd's Avenue, London EC3N 3AX; tel: 0171 488 9341; and Travelcare Ltd, 68 High Street, Chislehurst, Kent BR5 5AQ; tel: 0181 295 1234 or (freephone) 0800 181532.

MS SOCIETY CENTRES

Anyone who is looking for a UK holiday where they can be sure of finding all the facilities they need backed up with the right kind of service should know about the eight centres run by the Society. The holiday homes and respite care centres welcome guests with MS who want to get away for a break on their own. One or two can also accommodate family or friends or will be willing to suggest other places nearby where they can stay if required. Full details are in the booklet *Holidays For People With MS*, available from the Society, but here is a taster to whet your appetite:

- Brambles Respite Care Centre, Suffolk Close, Massetts Road, Horley, Surrey RH6 7DU; tel: 01293 784478.
  As well as twenty-eight single, ground floor rooms, there are two lounge areas, a conservatory, restaurant and bar plus a fully staffed physiotherapy/hydrotherapy unit. Other activities include reflexology, aromatherapy, art therapy, yoga and meditation and trained staff are available twenty-four hours a day.
- Helen Ley Home, Bericote Road, Blackdown, Leamington Spa, Warwickshire CV32 6QP; tel: 01926 313550.
  Set in the countryside, the purpose-built home has nineteen single and two twin rooms, together with a large lounge, sun lounge and dining room. Trained staff are on duty twenty-four hours a day, and the facilities are suitable for people with severe disabilities.
- Kenninghall MS Care Hotel, 13 Shakespeare Road, Worthing, West Sussex BN11 4AR; tel: 01903 238945.
  A family-style hotel with home-cooked food and six single and six twin-bedded rooms not far from the sea front and town centre. Fully staffed and equipped to cater for all levels of disability, this hotel is very popular – book early!

- The Richard Cave MS Holiday Home, c/o the MS Society in Scotland, 2a North Charlotte Street, Edinburgh EH2 4HR; tel: 0131 225 3600. Located in an eighteenth century Servite Convent in Leuchie, near North Berwick, it has room for twenty-two guests in single, double and triple-bedded rooms. The listed building has been fully modernized although still keeping its character, and is happy to welcome family and friends.

- Holmhill, c/o The MS Society in Scotland (address above). Up to fourteen guests at a time (including friends and relatives) can stay at the MS Holiday Centre at Grantown-on-Spey in the Highlands. There is a lounge, dining room with bar and a games room with exercise equipment and large screen tv/video. Full nursing care is provided, but only emergency staff are on call between 11 p.m. and 8 a.m.

- Orcombeleigh, 22 Douglas Avenue, Exmouth, Devon EX8 2HA; tel: 01395 272644.
  All the bedrooms have views over the sea, central heating, hot and cold water and their own tv. The home has a lounge with a sun terrace, bar and new dining room, plus a hydrotherapy pool and physiotherapy room with a resident physiotherapist. Guests can arrange to be picked up by ambulance from Exeter St David's station.

- Danygraig Respite Care Centre, Newton, Porthcawl, Mid Glamorgan CF36 5SR; tel: 0165678 2643.
  Set in attractive grounds on the outskirts of the resort of Porthcawl, the centre has twelve beds available through the Society. Facilities include a small hydrotherapy pool, Arjo and spa baths and a licensed bar.

- Woodlands Respite Care Centre, 120 Thief Lane, Hull Road, York YO1 3HU; tel: 01904 430600.
  Opened in 1991, the centre stands in wooded grounds within the city boundary. The twenty bedrooms have en

suite facilities equipped for any degree of disability and full twenty-four-hour nursing care is provided. There is a physiotherapy and hydrotherapy suite, a hairdressing salon and a bar, and excursions are arranged into York and the surrounding area.

Transport

Even if you are unable to use buses or underground trains, you may be able to use BR trains if the right kind of assistance is available. You need to check in advance with the stations concerned as to what is possible. Similarly, many taxi companies are happy to carry people with mobility problems given advance notice. The Dial-a-Ride service can be useful, but provision is patchy, so contact your local social services department to find out what's available in your area.

9

ORGANIZATIONS

THE MS SOCIETY

The Multiple Sclerosis Society of Great Britain and Northern Ireland, 25 Effie Road, London SW6 1EE; tel: 0171 610 7171.

The MS Society in Scotland, 2a North Charlotte Street, Edinburgh EH2 4HR; tel: 0131 225 3600.

Northern Ireland Office, 34 Annandale Avenue, Belfast BT7 3JJ; tel: 01232 644914.

e-mail: Info@mssociety.org.uk.

Web site: http://www.mssociety.org.uk.

Founded in 1953, the Society now has 60,000 members and offers help to anyone who has the condition, their families, friends and colleagues. It funds many of the medical research programmes – to the tune of £8 million annually, and the assets devoted to the service of people with MS total some £30 million, including residential and day centres, buses and ambulances.

In April 1996, the Society published *Reaching for the Stars*, its plan of campaign for the next five years, following extensive consultation with people with MS. Out of this, two major goals were identified:

- To offer more and better support for people with MS and their carers, and engage them as users and consumers.
- To ensure that everyone with MS has equal access to the Society's main services, wherever they live.

For most people, the first point of contact with the Society is through one of the main offices (see above), but there is also a network of 370 local branches throughout the country. Anyone can join either as a headquarters or a branch member (or both); subscription is a minimum of £3 a year (although any extra donation is always welcome) and some branches make a small additional charge.

Anyone can send for any of the Society's comprehensive range of free booklets and leaflets giving accurate and up-to-date information on everything from symptoms to diet and claiming benefits. For a full list, contact the London office. Members also receive the Society's magazine *MS Matters*, published six times a year.

There is a telephone helpline on 0171 371 8000 for general information and advice, (Monday to Friday, 10 a.m. to 4 p.m.) plus counselling lines in London 0171 222 3123 (24-hour); Midlands 0121 476 4229 and Scotland 0131 226 6573 (both 10 a.m. to 10 p.m.). These are answered by trained volunteers with personal experience of MS who are happy to talk to anyone with MS or their friends and families.

What is on offer at local branches will vary depending on the interests and needs of their members. However, all provide opportunities to meet other members in the area and their welfare officers can give advice and information, usually in the member's own home if required. They'll be well informed about local facilities and can often advise on obtaining benefits and help from social services departments. Branches vary in size from five to 400 members. Some run day centres, sometimes including the services of a physiotherapist, some have special groups or education sessions for people whose MS is newly diagnosed.

It's entirely up to you whether you contact your local branch or become a member; many people prefer to join as HQ members or only join their local branch after belonging to the Society for many years.

MS RESOURCE CENTRE LTD

4a Chapel Hill, Stansted, Essex, CM24 8AG; tel: 01279 817101.

The centre offers a wealth of information, advice and support on all aspects of MS to people with MS and their families, friends and colleagues.

In addition to providing advice and information to callers on the phone, they are willing to discuss personal problems but can also suggest how you can find a 'face-to-face' counsellor. As well as benefiting from their extensive bank of information, you can ask for details of other organizations and sources of information. To paraphrase the AA, if they don't know the answer to your question, they'll know someone who does. Contact the MSRC for details of your nearest centre. To become a subscriber costs £20.

- **Publications** The centre publishes a comprehensive range of information leaflets on a wide variety of MS-related topics, including complementary therapies, orthodox treatment, diet and a series under the overall title 'Bodycare'. They also produce *Pathways*, a quarterly newletter which is free to subscribers.

- **Booklist** A selection of useful books is available by post – write or ring for full details.
- **Benefitline** Ring the main number and ask to be put through for up-to-date and accurate information on your personal situation.
- **Researchline** Ring for the latest information and guidance on research into MS and new treatment (for subscribers only).

It's best to ring rather than write in the first instance if possible to discuss what help you need and how to go about getting it. The staff and volunteers are very approachable and sympathetic and keen to tailor the service they offer to meet the needs of each individual with MS, their families and friends.

MS THERAPY CENTRES

There are numerous centres around the country, the majority of which were formerly part of the network set up by ARMS, the MS charity which went bankrupt in 1992. Depending on their size and local arrangements, the centres offer complementary therapies of various kinds including physiotherapy, hyperbaric oxygen and dietary advice and some can provide counselling too.

Federation of MS Therapy Centres
Tel: 01234 325781 for information on your nearest centre.
Over seventy centres around the country.
Northern Association of MS Therapy Centres
Tel: 0161 872 3422
Association of Therapy Centres (Scotland)
Tel: 01382 566283. Over twelve centres in Scotland.

Lizzy: *'I was a founder member of what was originally an ARMS therapy centre. We had a wonderful physio who was*

170

really good at explaining the purpose of the various exercises. I used to do a kind of marching-on-the-spot which she called "running through the bracken", because she said it was like children making a new short-cut – making a new route for the CNS to pass messages more effectively. At first we just had chairs, but we gradually acquired more equipment and it was brilliant. Sadly, I can't go any more because they now have their own new building which is too far away for me to get to.'

MS (RESEARCH) CHARITABLE TRUST

Spirella Building, Letchworth, Herts SG6 4ET; tel: 01462 675613.

The Trust was set up in 1993 'to fund research into ways of improving the lives of people who have MS **now**, and to provide a more positive approach to the disease.' The research projects supported by the Trust are aimed at helping people with MS to manage their disease and developing much-needed therapies and strategies. The Trustees all have direct experience of MS, either through research, as carers or by having MS themselves. As a direct result of this personal involvement, they have recognized that many people are not given proper information and support at the time when they are most likely to need it – when their condition is first diagnosed. Part of their efforts are devoted to filling this gap, both for the person with MS and their family and friends. To this end, they have produced an excellent information pack, including summaries of therapies and approaches which may be helpful in dealing with the problems of MS, plus a useful list of contacts. Write to them at the above address; any donation you can afford to make towards their costs would be appreciated.

THE MYELIN PROJECT

4 Cammo Walk, Edinburgh EH4 8AN; tel: 0131 339 1316.

This is the UK arm of an international charity dedicated to 'accelerating life-saving research into the repair of the myelin sheath in demyelinating conditions such as leukodystrophies and multiple sclerosis'.

THE NERVE CENTRE

Mariner House, 62 Prince Street, Bristol BS1 4QD; tel: 0117 930 8642.

This is a charity which raises funds for research being conducted in the MS Unit of the Bristol Royal Infirmary. They keep a comprehensive database, and can give information and advice on many aspects of MS, including disability, mobility, benefits, home aids and adaptations and therapy. Trained telephone counsellors are available to listen and talk to people with MS and those close to them. They also produce a quarterly newsletter and other information sheets. Their service is free, although they would appreciate any donation you can afford to make towards their costs.

THE WORLD OF MS

http://www.ifmss.org.uk

The web site of the International Federation of MS Societies with links to the MS Society in the UK and similar organizations elsewhere in the world. As well as information on the societies, you can access the latest research findings, the most frequently asked questions about MS and links to other Internet sites on MS.

JOOLY'S JOINT

http://dspace.dial. pipex.com/town/square/ae218/

This is a free, worldwide webpal service, accessible via the Internet, for people living with MS. It was started in August 1995 by Julie Howell who's in her twenties and has had MS since 1992. As well as the contact service, Jooly's Joint also features Lotty's Lounge, where you can find stories, poems, questions and answers about MS and links to other MS sites on the worldwide web.

10

TOWARDS NEW TREATMENTS

New drugs

Until the first of the so-called beta interferon drugs was licensed for use in 1996, doctors could only try to treat the symptoms of MS. Nothing in their medical armoury had any effect on the underlying course of the disease. The development of a drug which, albeit in a limited way, could inhibit the disease process, is clearly important and encouraging. Neither this nor other treatments on the horizon promise a cure for MS, but nevertheless they represent a fundamental change in the landscape. Everyone now realizes that progress is being made and the resultant publicity has raised the profile of MS in the public mind. Pharmaceutical companies have recognized the potential of developing new treatments, and research programmes are under way all over the world. Work on potential new treatments is well advanced, and it is likely that one or more new drugs will become available within the near future. They will be prescribed through hospital neurology departments rather than GPs, so if you don't see a neurologist regularly, make a point of checking on the latest situation with your GP from time to time. He or she can then arrange for you to see a neurologist if required. You can also get an update on new treatments by ringing the MS Society helpline (see page 168).

As well as investigating specific compounds for their potential as therapy in MS, many researchers are studying the various physical changes which occur in the body of someone with MS and the reasons why they occur. There are many different approaches, looking at different factors involved in the development of MS.

In order for someone to develop MS, there must be a number of predisposing factors. Some researchers are looking at the genetic component to try and identify what exactly makes some people potentially vulnerable to MS while others aren't. This involves population, family and twins studies to try and work out who develops MS and what genetic factors may be significant. On a larger scale, work is being done on the geographical distribution of MS – why do people in some regions seem more likely to develop it than those living elsewhere? This might help to identify which environmental factors are important. Possible culprits being studied include diet, stress, gender and infectious agents such as viruses.

In another sphere of research, scientists are concentrating on learning more about exactly what happens to cause the destruction of the myelin sheath. Something must trigger the immune response which causes the damage – but what? It might well be certain viruses, but if so, we need to know which ones and exactly what effect they are having. We also need to understand why some people have an abnormal immune system response. For example, if scientists could work out why the T cells of the immune system are not under proper control in MS, they might be able to design methods of improving that control or turning off their unwanted action. As we saw in chapter 1, one of the malfunctions in the bodies of people with MS is that the so-called blood-brain barrier is breached, allowing attacking cells to reach the myelin sheath around the nerves of the CNS. By finding out why this happens, it might be possible to find ways of preventing it.

Other studies are looking at the nerves themselves, analysing mechanisms which damage the myelin sheath and what then happens to the exposed axons. Ultimately, this work could suggest ways of halting and/or repairing the damage.

Enormous amounts of effort and money are being put into research in all these areas and others in the hope that greater and more precise knowledge of what exactly is going on will open doors to new therapeutic approaches. Some experts suggest that there may eventually be more than one answer. In other words, different drugs might be developed to deal with different aspects of the problem of MS. Rather than a single 'cure', it might be that a combination of treatments is needed to beat it. It's also conceivable that different people might benefit from different treatments. While such treatments are not just around the corner, there is optimism that they will come in time, and the picture is no longer as blank as it was just a few years ago.

Meanwhile, advances are also being made in monitoring the effects of treatment and assessing damage more precisely, with different ways of interpreting the information provided by MRI scans. Enhanced MRI scanning methods give greatly increased sensitivity, and are particularly useful in assessing the effect of possible new treatments on brain lesions. This is of vital importance because of the difficulties of testing new pharmaceutical compounds. The unpredictability of MS and the relatively long time-scale needed to assess whether a treatment under test is showing real benefit make for slow progress. Sophisticated methods of MRI scanning can identify promising new agents more quickly so that further research can be directed towards those with real potential. Humans are the only creatures who get MS, although some animals do get related diseases, so scans are an essential tool in improving our understanding of MS.

Clinical trials

Testing new drugs is, inevitably, a slow and complicated process. They have to be shown to be safe, effective and without intolerable side effects. The only scientifically reliable way of assessing the effectiveness of a new treatment is the double-blind, placebo-controlled trial. People who are invited to take part in any trial will be selected on the basis of predetermined criteria – such as how long they have had MS, what type they have, age, sex and so on. Once the participants have been chosen, they will be divided into groups made up of people who are similar to one another in all respects important to that particular trial. Often there will be two groups, sometimes more, depending on what exactly is being studied. One group will always be given a 'placebo', an inert substitute for the drug being studied which is indistinguishable from the 'real thing' to everyone involved. So, for example, if the real treatment is given as daily injections of a clear fluid, the placebo will be given in exactly the same way. Sometimes, the group receiving the active compound will be subdivided again – with one section being given a higher and the other a lower dose. Neither the volunteers nor those giving the treatment will know who is in which group. The effects of the real treatment and the placebo will be closely monitored, and those doing the monitoring will also be 'blind' as to who's getting what.

The groups are usually quite large so as to give a statistically significant result, and trials frequently continue for up to two years. Clearly, it is especially important when testing treatments for MS to have a relatively large group and to continue the study for a considerable length of time because of the natural variations in the course of the condition between both individual people and in any one person over a period of time.

Before the trial starts, the researchers will have decided what exactly they are looking for – it may be that the main objective is to assess whether the treatment has an effect on the number of relapses, for example. This will influence the way the trial is designed. In the trial of beta interferon 1b (see pages 180–3), for example, the effect on relapse rate was the so-called 'primary outcome measure', and although some conclusions were drawn about the drug's effect on developing disability, further trials are now needed which have disability as the primary end point.

Disability is commonly assessed both when recruiting and during trials by means of a scale known as the Kurtzke disability status scale (or DSS). Various factors are rated by numbers – for example, when assessing walking, 0 is normal, 6 means you use a stick, 8 means you use a wheelchair and so on. It is by no means a perfect method but it has been widely used for very many years.

If you are ever invited to take part in such a trial, the organizers are required to explain all this to you quite clearly, including what the treatment involves, how long it is likely to last and what will be asked of you. It's important to bear in mind that you will not know whether you are receiving the treatment under test and, even if you are, there is no guarantee that it will have any beneficial effect on your health.

AT THE STARTING GATE

Only one of the new treatments which has an effect on the course of MS has been licensed for use at the time of writing, but others are expected to become available very soon. Check with your neurologist or one of the MS charities for the latest situation.

Interferons

These are proteins which the body manufactures naturally. They influence the workings of the immune system, stimulating and suppressing different components as circumstances demand. There are different types of interferon, and the important ones in this context are interferon-gamma and interferon-beta. The former seems to be implicated in the attack on, and destruction of, the myelin sheath, while interferon-beta appears to interrupt this activity. The interferons used in the new drug formulations are produced by genetic engineering techniques from one of two sources. Beta interferon 1b is made from a bacterial cell and this is the type used in Schering's Betaferon. Beta interferon 1a, made from mammal cells, is used in the new treatments from Serono and Biogen. Betaferon has been shown in a two-year, multi-centre trial to have some effect on relapsing/remitting MS in the early stages. The study found that those people who were given beta interferon 1b had approximately one third fewer relapses than the control group given a placebo, and their relapses were also less severe. MRI scans showed that the treated patients had fewer visible lesions in the CNS after two years in the trial than they had when it began, compared to a 20 per cent increase in the untreated patients.

These findings are obviously good news, but there are qualifications. So far, treatment with beta interferon 1b has not been shown to have any effect on the development of disability. The people in the trial had relapsing/remitting MS and were not badly affected at the time they joined when they were required to walk 100 metres without any aid or rest. As yet, no studies have been published on the effects of beta interferon 1b on progressive MS and it is not expected to hold much promise for those with severe disabilities.

The treatment, which was given by injection every other day, was not without side effects. The commonest problems were flu-like symptoms and inflammation at the injection site, and some people also experienced periods of depression. Usually these reactions subsided in the course of treatment. Around 40 per cent of people developed antibodies against the drug, which meant that it then stopped being effective. The proportion of people reacting in this way could be expected to increase with long-term treatment.

Some neurologists are not convinced that the benefits of

the drug outweigh the disadvantages, especially in view of the fact that it does not seem to slow the development of disability. Some also believe that their patients would do better to wait a little longer until treatment based on beta interferon 1a become available in the belief that this may also show some effect on the development of disability and be less likely to trigger the production of antibodies.

The picture is complicated by the fact that treating one person for a year with Betaferon costs £10,000. This is also likely to be the case with the 1a drugs when they are licensed. Each local health authority has to decide whether beta interferon will be funded for people within their area in discussion with local specialists. The result is that whether you will be eligible for treatment may depend in part on where you live. In those areas where the treatment is available, whether an individual is eligible is decided on the basis of strict clinical criteria and whether their doctors think they can benefit. However, there is naturally some concern that such decisions may be unduly influenced by financial rather than purely clinical criteria. There are reports that in some areas, people with MS have been asked to justify why they should be given treatment costing £10,000 per year in the hope of cutting their annual relapses from three a year to two when the same money could buy several hip replacement operations, for example. Should you feel that you are being refused treatment on purely financial grounds, despite meeting the clinical criteria and wanting to take it, you may well decide to put up a fight. Those with the necessary energy and determination can exert quite a lot of pressure not only on doctors, but through their local paper, MP, the area health authority and the Department of Health. You could also contact the MS Resource Centre for advice on tactics. It may or may not work, but the more the voice of people with MS is heard in their own interests, the more notice the rest of the world is likely to take.

Licenses for drugs based on the other type of beta interferon are imminent. The trial of Biogen's Avonex – beta interferon 1a – not only reduced the relapse rate by a third and reduced the number of active brain lesions visible on MRI scans, it also slowed the rate at which disability progressed. This is an important advance and the first time a drug has been shown to do this. One and two year progression rates were delayed by around 40 per cent.

The treatment involved one injection a week. As with the beta interferon 1b trial, 1a was tested on people who'd had relapsing/remitting MS for at least a year and whose degree of disability was relatively mild. Similar results have been obtained from trials on the other beta interferon 1a – Serono Rebif. At the time of writing, it looks as if Avonex will be licensed before Rebif, although neither should be very far off.

Copolymer 1

A trial carried out on people with relapsing/remitting MS showed that the relapse rate in those given daily injections of copolymer 1 was reduced by around 29 per cent. There was a slight reduction in the progression of disability, but none of the people in the study had yet experienced any serious difficulties in this respect. Side effects were minor, didn't last long and, in any case, only affected a small proportion of those taking part. As yet, it is not known whether copolymer 1 will benefit people with more serious disabilities or those with a progressive form of MS. At the moment, the jury is still out on this drug and it is not yet clear whether it is likely to become available in the immediate future.

11

COMMON QUESTIONS ASKED ABOUT MS

I think I may have MS, but my doctor says she can't be sure. How can I find out?

It's likely that you have experienced one or more symptoms which could possibly be due to MS, but which might also have some other, unrelated cause. When there is doubt doctors often prefer to wait to see whether a person has a subsequent attack which might confirm the initial suspicion of MS before arranging further tests. If you are now well again, your doctor may feel that there is no point in sending you to see a neurologist unless or until you have further symptoms. Some people with MS have no further problems after the initial attack or remain well for many years afterwards. If, on the other hand, you have had several bouts of unexplained symptoms or if you are not now fully recovered, it's worth going back and asking your doctor to refer you to hospital for further investigations. Some doctors say nothing to patients whom they believe to have MS in an attempt to protect them from the truth, not realizing that this is often more difficult to handle than a correct diagnosis.

Why did I get MS?

The reasons why some people get MS are not fully understood, but a combination of factors must be involved. It is more common in women than men and in people who are brought up in the temperate rather than the tropical zones of the world. It also seems that there is a genetic element, in that some people are born with a susceptibility to the condition, although by no means all of them will actually develop it. One current theory is that the actual disease may be triggered in susceptible people by a virus, possibly lying dormant in the body, but no such virus or viruses have yet been specifically identified. At the moment, no one can tell you exactly why you developed MS. However, it is not the result of anything you did (or failed to do) and you could not have prevented it.

Could the doctors have made a mistake in diagnosing my MS?

While there is no single test that can prove definitively that anyone has MS, a history of your symptoms taken with the results of a range of other tests will usually give a clear-cut diagnosis. If you have had a number of symptoms at different times which fit with a diagnosis of MS plus an MRI scan and other neurological procedures, it is very unlikely that a mistake has been made. You need to talk over your worries and ask for a proper explanation of the diagnosis you've been given. The best person to see is probably the doctor who gave you the diagnosis or, if you prefer, you could ask your GP.

My neurologist has said I need a course of steroids – aren't they dangerous?

Steroids can sometimes help to ease symptoms or reduce the severity and length of a relapse. They are often effective when given early in the course of MS, especially if the person has symptoms of optic neuritis. As well as their major role of reducing inflammation they also damp down the immune system. However, like all powerful drugs they have side effects which may be serious if the steroids are not used with care. At one time, these risks were not as well recognized as they are today and some people did experience very serious problems. Your neurologist will know how to use them safely. A more significant problem than potential side effects is the fact that steroids do not always work for everyone.

Will my children inherit MS from me?
You do not carry MS in your genes in the same way that, for example, you might carry a genetically transmitted condition such as cystic fibrosis or haemophilia. So no child of yours can inherit MS from you. He or she may, however, face an increased risk of developing the disease as a result of having a parent with MS. Nevertheless, many other factors are involved in determining who does or does not develop MS, and an inherited susceptibility is only one of them. Even the identical twin of someone with MS who shares precisely the same genes will not necessarily develop the condition. Other factors have to play their part, too, in order for someone to develop MS.

Can stress make MS worse?
This is a complicated question and the answer depends partly on how you define stress. Events or situations which put you under pressure so that you feel you can't cope can result in chemical changes in your body. The so-called stress hormones do have an effect on your immune response so it's possible stress could have an indirect effect on your MS. Many people with MS say that their symptoms are triggered

or made worse by severe stress. It's also quite common to find that your legs 'seize up' when you're trying to get out of someone's way or do something very quickly. You could say that this type of situation is really one of minor panic or anxiety, rather than stress. Although there are some things which almost everyone regards as stressful – such as losing their job or a bereavement – others will produce different responses in different people. Deadlines, for example, are only stressful to some people at certain times, while others regard them as a necessary stimulus and a positive element in their lives. Finding the best ways to handle stress can't help but improve your overall well-being, since you can't avoid it altogether. Relaxation classes, yoga, aromatherapy and counselling have all been found by some people to help them cope better with stress.

Will pregnancy and childbirth make my MS worse?
Many women actually find that they have fewer problems than usual with their MS while they are pregnant. One theory is that this may be because your body produces hormones which have the effect of mild steroids during this time. You may like to ask your neurologist's advice as to whether this is a good time for you to plan a pregnancy if he or she knows you and your MS well. As far as the birth is concerned, nearer the time you'll need to discuss what kind of delivery you are going to have with your obstetrician and neurologist in case your MS symptoms put any limits on the options available to you. A woman with muscle weakness may need to have a planned Caesarean delivery or specialized anaesthetic care to make an epidural safe. There does seem to be an increased risk of exacerbations of MS during the months immediately after having a baby. Around one in five women find this happens but it is unpredictable. In any case,

there is no evidence that your MS will be any worse in the long term than if you had not had children.

I want to fight against MS, but my family think life would be easier if I gave in to it more. Won't that just mean it gets worse more quickly?
A lot of people with MS believe that you must 'use it or lose it', while others feel there's no point in wasting energy on battles they can't win. Whether you choose to fight and on what grounds is a personal decision. For some people, fighting means ignoring their MS and its effects on them and trying to carry on exactly as they did before. A refusal to make any concessions can be part of making it clear to everyone (and even to yourself) that you are still the same person. Unfortunately, it can sometimes seem to other people that you are simply being stubborn in not acknowledging that there are some things you can no longer do well or at all. Instead of taking up positions which are poles apart, it might help if everyone could see that it really doesn't have to be a straight choice between this kind of fighting and giving in. Some people describe their way of fighting as learning to 'cooperate' with their MS symptoms – planning activities so that they don't get too exhausted, getting organized so that avoidable frustration is reduced and finding ways around problems instead of trying to charge straight over them. 'Giving in' in the sense of recognizing and adapting to meet reality can't make your MS worse. It will not affect the amount of neurological damage you experience nor how quickly it occurs. It doesn't mean sinking back into your chair and refusing to engage with life ever again. You may also need to think about the ways in which your priorities differ from those of your family and discuss this with them if possible. Your relatives may have a

point in saying that life would be easier if you battled less, but perhaps they mean easier for them rather than (or as well as) for you.

Can I do anything to stave off a relapse?

Some people with relapsing/remitting MS say that they become aware a few days before a relapse that it's about to happen. There's usually nothing very definite, just a subtle shift in feeling – perhaps greater irritability or increased emotional sensitivity or a sense that life is somehow getting on top of them. If they respond to these sensations by resting and putting off all non-essential activity for a few days, the relapse may be less severe or last for a shorter time. There's no guarantee that this will always work, but it may be worth a try. If, on the other hand, they ignore the warning signs and try to carry on as usual, they may get away with it for a while. Eventually, however, they experience new symptoms or old ones become more pronounced and they have no choice but to slow down and wait for the exacerbation to pass. Most people feel worse when they experience a bout of fatigue. Sometimes, this comes on out of the blue, but it can also happen when you are pushing yourself hard, especially when you're not getting enough sleep or are expending a lot of physical or mental energy. You may feel it is worth trying to pace yourself so that you can build quieter patches into your life as and when you need them. Eating the right kind of diet and paying attention to your overall health will boost your general sense of well-being and are worthwhile in themselves. It may be appropriate to consult a doctor if you find a particular symptom is troubling you more than usual to see whether anything can be done to ease it. If the relapse comes despite all your efforts, you may have little choice but to live through it as best you can, although in some circumstances, a course of steroids may be helpful.

I've heard that a gluten-free diet can help – is this true?
While there are people who are sure that following this kind of diet has brought about a remission of their MS, there is no scientific evidence whatsoever to back this up. Nor is there any logical reason why eating foods containing gluten – found in products made from wheat – should make MS worse. This, together with the fact that a gluten-free diet involves a lot of self-denial, suggests that the disadvantages far outweigh any possible benefits. In practical terms, avoiding everyday foods such as bread, pasta, pastry, cakes and biscuits – not to mention most sauces and many other processed foods – isn't at all easy. You would do much better to follow a healthy, balanced diet which includes lots of fresh fruit and vegetables, fish and unrefined carbohydrates, such as wholemeal bread and pasta, and foods high in polyunsaturated rather than saturated (animal) fats. For most people, food is a source of pleasure as well as fuel and it's pointless to deprive yourself of this unless you have to.

Should I take vitamin or mineral supplements?
Nutritionists stress that the best way to get all the vitamins and minerals you need is from your diet. In their natural form, they seem to confer benefits which you don't get by taking them separately in the form of pills or capsules. Unless you know what you're doing, it is theoretically possible to take too much of some vitamins, while others will simply pass straight through your system if they're not needed. What's more, you can end up spending a fortune without doing yourself much good in return. Sometimes, difficulties with swallowing or other problems may mean you can't

manage to eat the right kind of diet, and in this situation, supplements may have a useful role to play. However, rather than simply dosing yourself, you should get advice from your GP or a dietitian on what you need to take and in what amounts.

I'd like to try some complementary therapy, but I don't know how to find out more about what's available and where to go for treatment.
There is an enormous choice available and you need to do some research to find out what each involves and which, if any, will suit you best. A good starting point might be to think about what you are hoping to get out of complementary therapy. While none can offer a cure or even guarantee any improvement in symptoms, they can sometimes bring some relief and increase your overall sense of well-being. Some, such as aromatherapy, are very enjoyable in themselves, others, such as acupuncture, can be energizing and many are particularly good at easing stress and tension. It is worth remembering, however, that in theory anyone can set themselves up as a complementary therapist without any checks being made, so you have to choose your practitioner carefully. The organizations listed on pages 206–9 are worth contacting for individual therapies and you can also get information from the Insitute for Complementary Medicine (see page 208). The many MS therapy centres around the country are also useful sources of advice and some also offer some forms of complementary therapies on their premises. Contact one of the organizations listed on page 202 to find your nearest centre. Depending on where you live, you may also find that some therapies are available at or through your GP's surgery or the health centre so it's worth making enquiries. If you approach a therapist who isn't working

within the NHS, don't forget to ask about costs and how many sessions you should expect to have before experiencing any benefits.

I saw a TV programme about Cari Loder's treatment – where can I get it?
The treatment consists of three elements: an antidepressant, an amino acid and injections of vitamin B12. Since two of the three are only available on prescription, you have to have the support of a doctor, who would normally be your GP. There are two major obstacles, however. One is that details of the antidepressant and amino acid are no longer being made public pending the start of trials of the treatment by a pharmaceutical company. The other is that many doctors are, in any case, reluctant to cooperate because of doubts about its usefulness and concerns about possible side effects. Should the trial results of Cari Loder's treatment show positive benefits, with no serious side effects, you can be sure that it will be front-page news.

My MS was diagnosed three years ago, and so far I have not had any major problems, but should I start planning now about how I'm going to manage later on if I become more disabled?
According to the best available estimates, only one in four people with MS will eventually develop serious disabilities. In theory this should be reassuring, but it doesn't help very much when no one can tell you for sure whether or not you are likely to be one of them. There are a few considerations which may be a guide to what lies ahead. Possible pointers might include the age at which you first had symptoms, the nature of those symptoms and the length of time between a first and subsequent attack. As ever with MS, what is true in

general is often not so in particular. Your case is quite likely to be an exception – as is virtually anyone else's – so doctors will probably be unwilling to offer an opinion about the likely progression of your MS. As far as forward planning is concerned, you may be someone who prefers to anticipate and prepare. If so, there can be no harm in thinking about what arrangements you might want to make for particular eventualities. While it wouldn't make much sense, for instance, to buy a wheelchair now if you are still pretty mobile, it might be useful to find out where your nearest Disabled Living Centre is or even to visit it to see what might come in useful later. Some people say it has helped them to imagine the worst and work out how they would cope if it happened, but others would see this as unnecessarily gloomy or pessimistic. Do what feels right for you.

My neurologist doesn't seem to be able to offer me anything – is it worth keeping on seeing him?
It depends on whether you feel that you want something from him or might be able to benefit from his knowledge and experience were he more forthcoming. On the other hand, you may feel that you're coping with your MS reasonably well and need nothing from the medical world for the moment. Either way, just turning up for routine appointments which yield nothing much of interest to either of you is pretty pointless. You may decide therefore to give yourself a break for a while at least. If you don't want to give up, why not try and see whether you can't get more out of your next encounter? If you have particular symptoms which are troubling you, make sure you get an opportunity to say so and ask whether anything can be done. Do you need to see another specialist for further

investigations and/or treatment – such as a urologist if you have bladder problems, for example? Ask about physiotherapy, new treatments, pain relief, counselling – anything you would like to know about. You might get little back, but with luck you might trigger a more valuable discussion from which you emerge with more knowledge at the least and more action if appropriate. If all this fails and you still feel you're not getting anywhere with this particular doctor, ask your GP whether he or she could refer you to another neurologist instead.

Should I tell everyone I've got MS – I don't want them to treat me differently?

There's no 'should' about it; it's up to you. Most people start by telling partners and members of their immediate family or a few friends. Others limit the knowledge to those they can't avoid telling and don't even tell close family or friends, at least to begin with. Some, probably a minority, mention that they have MS quite easily to anyone by way of information or explanation whenever it seems appropriate. Whatever line you choose to take, you're sure to be in for a lot of surprises, and possibly a few disappointments too. Probably everyone with MS has experienced strange and unpredictable reactions from people they thought they knew well. You really can't be completely sure how anyone will deal with the news of your MS until you try telling them. In any case, it will take most people some time and quite a lot of explanation before they have any clear idea of what it actually means. You may well have to educate them about MS at the same time as you're educating yourself. Whatever you do, it may be impossible to prevent some people treating you differently, which can be galling even when it's well-intentioned. Sometimes the difference is quite subtle – a friend who might once have been keen to keep you out late suddenly starts telling you it's your bedtime at midnight, for example. There's no easy way to handle this kind of thing or to avoid it altogether, but if you're lucky it may be balanced by some nice surprises too. You may hope that other people will take their cue from you or instinctively know what you want from them. Sometimes this will happen, but you may sometimes have to spell things out. Until or unless you are sure that you do want everyone to know, you have a perfect right to be selective about whom you tell.

Am I entitled to an orange badge for my car?

An orange badge will allow you or the person driving you to park in places where this would normally be forbidden or restricted and in special disabled parking bays. This can be a big convenience because it usually means you can park nearer to where you want to go and you shouldn't ever get wheelclamped – although the police might tow your car away if it's causing an obstruction. You apply for a badge through your local authority. You should get one automatically if you are receiving the higher rate mobility component of the disability allowance and in certain other circumstances, or if you have a 'permanent and substantial disability which causes inability to walk or very consider-able difficulty in walking'. This last condition can ob-viously be problematic for some people with MS whose mobility is variable. If you can walk reasonably well at some times but not at others, you should go by your 'worst case' situation. The badge can also be used by someone who is driving on your behalf – to pick you up or on the way back from dropping you off, for example. The rules on exactly where you may park and for how long may vary slightly from one area to another, so make sure you check the situation in an unfamiliar locality, although wardens are often sympathetic if you err by mistake! The badge may be free although local authorities are allowed to charge up to £2 for issuing one.

I'd like to talk to someone to try and sort out my feelings – where can I find a good counsellor?

A few hospital neurology departments and some GPs may have direct access to a counsellor, or be able to recommend one, but otherwise you will probably have to find someone for yourself. The MS Society runs a telephone counselling service and the MS Resource Centre may be able to recommend someone locally; you'll find details on page 201. Some of the local MS Therapy Centres also provide the services of a counsellor; you'll need to ring to find your nearest one and then contact them for more information. You'll find the contact numbers to ring for details of your nearest centre on page 202. You can get a list of counsellors who are members of the British Association of Counselling by writing to BAC, 7 Regent Place, Rugby, Warks CV21 2PJ, tel: 01788 550899. It may take you a while to find the right person for you. Relatively few counsellors have specific knowledge about MS and the problems it can bring, although this doesn't always matter if you find someone you can relate to well. However, if you and the counsellor feel some specialized information would be helpful, he or she can get some unpublished notes for professional counsellors who are working with people with MS from Julia Segal, CMH MS Unit, Central Middlesex Hospital, Acton Lane, London NW10 7NS; tel: 0181 453 2337. Julia is one of the few counsellors who specializes in working in this field and is part of the team at the hospital's rehabilitation centre. The unit will accept referrals from GPs anywhere in the country. You obviously have to pay to see a private counsellor, and fees vary. Many counsellors are happy to arrange an initial consultation to see whether you suit each other, and this will also give you the opportunity to discuss how many sessions you are likely to need and the costs. Once you've made the initial decision to seek counselling, it is worth spending time finding the right person and discussing what you hope to get out of the consultations before you commit yourself.

I've had to give up work. How can I find out what benefits I can claim?

Some of the benefits to which you may be entitled are specifically for people with disabilities while others depend on your general circumstances. Claiming one does not necessarily mean you can't claim others, so it's important to make sure you don't miss out. Any income, savings or other assets will need to be taken into consideration for those benefits which are means-tested, such as income support, housing benefit and council tax benefit. For others, your financial situation is less important, although it may be taken into consideration in some instances. Your National Insurance record is relevant for so-called 'contributory benefits'; these include unemployment and incapacity benefit. Many people with MS are also entitled to some 'non-contributory' benefits, such as the disability living allowance and attendance allowance. The system is run by the Department of Social Security (DSS) through the Benefits Agency and you can get general advice and information leaflets from them by phone, although they can't advise on individual cases or specifics. You can ring the free Benefit Enquiry Line which specializes in benefits for people with disabilities on 0800 882200; 0800 220674 in Northern Ireland. Freeline Social Security 0800 666555 will give general advice on all benefits. The benefits 'bible', *The Disability Rights Handbook* (see page 159), suggests that you ask the advisor to check and explain to you what the relevant guidance manual says about your situation. It also points out that both these lines are confidential and nothing you ask or say will go into your file. The MS Society also publishes various information leaflets on the benefits system; write to them or ring the helpline for more details (see pages 167–9). No one should hesitate or feel embarrassed about making sure they claim everything to which they are entitled.

Where can I find out about gadgets and adaptations to my home that would make it easier for me to remain independent?
Probably the best person to discuss this with is an occupational therapist who can be contacted through your local social services department. He or she will have a good knowledge of what's available and will help you to match the equipment or adaptations to suit your requirements. Some items can be borrowed on long-term loan from social services or the NHS. If you're considering buying any equipment or gadgets, it's always worth seeing them yourself and ideally giving them a try at home before spending your own money. You should be able to make an appointment to visit a local Disabled Living Centre where you can see and try a wide range of equipment. Contact the Disabled Living Centres Council, 1st Floor, Winchester House, 11 Cranmer Road, London SW9 6EJ for a list. Local social services may provide services or alterations to your home on the basis of an assessment of your needs. The local office is the place to start or your occupational therapist should be

able to advise you. Sometimes, grants may be available to help pay for modifications to the home of a person with disabilities – building a ramp to facilitate access, for example – and these are means-tested. These are administered through the local authority and your occupational therapist will be able to give you more information.

ADDRESS BOOK

MS Information And Support

ACT (Alliance for Cannabis Therapeutics)
PO Box CR14
Leeds LS7 4XG
Fax: 01132 371000

MS (Research) Charitable Trust
Spirella Building
Letchworth
Herts SG6 4ET
Tel: 01462 675613

MS Resource Centre
4a Chapel Hill
Stansted
Essex CM24 8AG
Tel: 01279 817101

MS Society
25 Effie Road
London SW6 1EE
Tel: 0171 610 7171

Scottish office:
2a North Charlotte Street
Edinburgh EH2 4HR
Tel: 0131 225 3600
N. Ireland office:
24 Annadale Avenue
Belfast BT7 3JJ
Tel: 01232 644914

MS Therapy Centres
Federation of MS Therapy Centres
Tel: 01234 325781
Association of Therapy Centres (Scotland)
Tel: 01382 566283
Northern Association of MS Therapy Centres
Tel: 0161 872 3422

The Nerve Centre
Mariner House
62 Prince Street
Bristol BS1 4QD
Tel: 0117 930 8642

Counselling

British Association for Counselling
7 Regent Place
Rugby
Warks CV21 2PJ
Tel: 01738 550899

Relate
Herbert Gray College
Little Church Street
Rugby
Warks CV21 3AP
Tel: 01788 550899

SPOD (The Association to Aid the Sexual and Personal
Relationships of People with a Disability)
286 Camden Road
London N7 0BJ
Tel: 0171 607 8851

Practical information and advice

Association of Disabled Professionals
170 Benton Hill
Horbury
Wakefield WF4 5HW
Tel: 01924 270335

Carers National Association
20–25 Glasshouse Yard
London EC1A 4JS
Tel: 0171 490 8818

Continence Foundation
2 Doughty Street
London WC1N 2PH
Tel: 0171 213 0050

Disability Alliance
Universal House
88-94 Wentworth Street
London E1 7SA
Tel: 0171 247 8776

Holiday Care Service
2nd Floor
Imperial Buildings
Victoria Road
Horley
Surrey RH6 9PZ
Tel: 01293 774535

Opportunities for People with Disabilities
1 Bank Buildings
Princes Street
London EC2R 8EU
Tel: 0171 726 4961

RADAR (The Royal Association for Disability and
Rehabilitation)
12 City Forum
250 City Road
London EC1V 8AF
Tel: 0171 250 3222

Mobility

Banstead Mobility Centre
Damson Way
Orchard Hill
Queen Mary's Avenue
Carshalton
Surrey SM5 4NR
Tel: 0181 770 1151

BSM Central Mobility Unit
Tel: 0181 540 8262

Department of Transport Mobility Advice and
Vehicle Information Centre
TRL
Crowthorne
Berks RG45 6AU

Disability Equipment Register
4 Chatterton Road
Yate
Bristol BS17 4BJ
Tel: 01454 318818

Disabled Drivers Association
Ashwellthorpe
Norfolk NR16 1EX
Tel: 01508 489449

Disabled Living Centres Council
1st Floor
Winchester House
11 Cranmer Road
London SW9 6EJ
Tel: 0171 820 0567

Mobility Information Service
Unit 2a
Atcham Industrial Estate
Upton Magna
Shrewsbury SY4 4UG
Tel: 01743 761889

Motability
Goodman House
Station Approach
Harlow
Essex CM20 2ET
Tel: 01279 635666

Complementary therapies

Acupuncture Association
34 Alderney Street
London SW1V 4EC
Tel: 0171 834 1012

Aromatherapy Organizations Council
Tel: 01455 615466

British Acupuncture Association and Register
34 Alderney Street
London SW1V 4EU
Tel: 0171 834 1012

British Acupuncture Council
Tel: 0181 964 0222

British Chiropractic Association
Premier House
10 Greycoat Place
London SW1P 1SD
Tel: 0171 222 8866

British Homoeopathic Association
27a Devonshire Street
London W1N 1RJ
0171 935 2163

British Society of Medical and Dental Hypnosis
Tel: 0181 905 4342

The General Council and Register of Osteopaths
56 London Street
Reading
Berks RG1 4SQ
Tel: 01734 576585

Institute for Complementary Medicine
Unit 15
Tavern Quay
Commercial Centre
Rope Street
London SE16 1TX
Tel: 0171 237 5165

International Federation of Aromatherapists
Stamford House
2–4 Chiswick High Road
London W4 1TH
Tel: 0181 742 2605

International Federation of Reflexology
76-8 Edridge Road
Croydon
Surrey CR0 1EF
Tel: 0181 667 9458

London College of Massage
5 Newman Passage
London W1P 3PF
Tel: 0171 323 3574

The National Federation of Spiritual Healers
Old Manor Farm Studio
Church Street
Sunbury on Thames
Middlesex TW16 6RG
Tel: 01932 783164

National Institute of Medical Herbalists
56 Longbrook Street
Exeter EX4 6AH

The Shiatsu Society
14 Oakdene Road
Redhill
Surrey RH1 6BT
Tel: 01737 767896

Yoga for Health Foundation
Ickwell Bury
Biggleswade
Beds SG8 9EF
Tel: 01767 627271

INDEX

Access to Work 161
ACT *see* Alliance for Cannabis Therapeutics
acupressure 61
acupuncture 60–61
  associations 206, 207
aids and adaptations 17, 136, 148, 151, 156–8, 199–200
alcohol 77–8
Alliance for Cannabis Therapeutics (ACT) 80–81, 201
Amantadine 52
amino acid 82, 193
anaesthetics 148, 149
antidepressants 46–8, 82, 193
appetite 44, 76
arachnidonic acid 75
ARMS 170–71
aromatherapy 63–4, 188
Aromatherapy Organizations Council 207
arsenic 4
Association of Disabled Professionals 161, 203
Association of Therapy Centres, Scotland 202
Avonex 183
axons 8, 177

baby, having 145–9, 188–9
Baclofen 46
balance, poor 15, 20, 53, 78, 79, 147
Banstead Mobility Centre 155, 205
belladonna 4
benefits 136, 151, 158–60, 168, 169, 172, 198–9
  telephone lines 159, 170, 198–9
Benefits Agency 159, 198
beta interferon
  1a 181, 182, 183
  1b 175, 179, 181–2
Betaferon 181, 182
Biogen 181, 183
bladder 12, 14, 24, 45, 48–50, 66, 79, 81
blind spots 20
blindness 15; *see also* visual disturbances
blood–brain barrier 8, 177
botulinum 51
bowel 14, 24, 50–51
brain 7, 8, 10, 18, 23, 26
breastfeeding 148
British Association for Counselling 197, 203
British Homoeopathic Association 66, 207

British School of Motoring (BSM) Mobility Unit 155, 205
British Society of Medical and Dental Hypnosis 68, 207
burning sensations 25, 47

cannabis 79–81
car 154–6
carbamazepine 48
carbohydrates 75–6, 191
Carers National Association 203
catheterization 49, 81
central nervous system (CNS) 10, 13, 22, 171, 177
cerebro-spinal fluid 8, 32
childbirth 148, 188–9; *see also* baby, having
children
  developing MS 15
  effect of parent's MS on 118–23
chiropractic 69
Citizens Advice Bureaux 160
clamminess 21–2
clumsiness 14, 15, 20; *see also* co-ordination
CNS *see* central nervous system
cognitive symptoms 18; *see also* memory problems; mental acuity
cold, as a trigger 139–40
colds 144
community care 152–3
community health services 158
complementary therapies 6, 57–8, 192–3, 206–9; *see also specific types of therapy*
concentration problems 18, 27, 78
constipation 24, 51
continence 12, 14, 24, 45, 48–50, 158
  advisors 50, 51, 158
Continence Foundation 204
cool suits 139
co-ordination, loss of 14, 20, 53, 78; *see also* clumsiness
Copolymer 1 183–4
corn oil 75
corticosteroids 43–6; *see also* steroids
counselling 36, 47, 92, 100–102, 169, 170, 197–8, 202–3
  telephone lines 168, 172, 197
cystitis 24; *see also* urinary infections

dancing 141
demyelination 8–9, 13, 22, 23, 138

211